LIVING ON BORROWED TIME
Life with Cystic Fibrosis

Debbie Pitts

Bloomington, IN 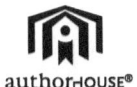 Milton Keynes, UK

authorHOUSE®

AuthorHouse™
1663 Liberty Drive, Suite 200
Bloomington, IN 47403
www.authorhouse.com
Phone: 1-800-839-8640

AuthorHouse™ UK Ltd.
500 Avebury Boulevard
Central Milton Keynes, MK9 2BE
www.authorhouse.co.uk
Phone: 08001974150

This book is a work of non-fiction. Unless otherwise noted, the author and the publisher make no explicit guarantees as to the accuracy of the information contained in this book and in some cases, names of people and places have been altered to protect their privacy.

First published by AuthorHouse 1/16/2007

ISBN: 978-1-4259-4574-9 (sc)

Printed in the United States of America
Bloomington, Indiana

This book is printed on acid-free paper.

More than 30,000 people in the U.S. today have a hereditary lung disease called Cystic Fibrosis. Most babies born with this disease never live beyond their teen years. Those who do, have a very difficult life. CF is not curable at this time. Better genetic tests and earlier diagnosis are helping the numbers of survivers to rise. This information is available from the National Cystic Fibrosis Foundation.

There are booklets and pamplets available about CF. But there are only two paperback books out about real people who lived and died with this terrible disease. One book is about an eight year old girl, the other book tells of a girl who lived to be twenty-one. Wouldn't it be great to have a book available for older patients with CF and the general public to read?

I have Cystic Fibrosis myself, and I am thirty-one years old. When searching for books on older people with CF, I found none. Only the two books I mentioned were available. The CF foundation thought that my writing a book on the subject would be great.

My book tells how I have struggled to live from day to day since my being diagnosed at six months of age. So you know I have lived a long time with this disease. It hasn't been easy.

I have enclosed several pages so that you can see what I mean. I have spoken to many medical students, doctors, nurses, and respiratory therapist about this subject. They all feel like my book could be useful to many people just starting in the medical field, as well as newly diagnosed patients and parents of CF babies. I hope you feel the same way.

If you would like to see more of my book, please feel free to contact me at your earliest convenience. I hope to hear from you soon.

Sincerely,

Debbie Pitts

LIVING ON BORROWED TIME: LIFE WITH CYSTIC FIBROSIS

This is my life story about living with a serious lung disease called Cystic Fibrosis. I am an older CF patient. I am one of the lucky ones; most babies born with this genetic killer disease die before they reach their teens. Cystic Fibrosis takes away any dreams of a normal lifestyle for anyone diagnosed with it. Since so many patients die young, it is unusual to meet older people with CF. I am thirty-one years old. People say I am very lucky to still be alive. The quality of my life makes me wonder if I am so lucky or not. I have a very difficult life to say the least.

This book is dedicated to the love of my life, Jimmy. Without his love and support, I could not make it from day to day. He is a precious and important part of my life.

To my entire family that I love very much – Thank you all for caring so much about me. You all have helped me through some very rough times.

And to Dr. Brevard Haynes and his nurse Teresa, the respiratory staff, and other nurses at Saint Thomas Hospital, my deepest gratitude for all the wonderful care that I get from you.

Finally, I want to dedicate this story of love and sacrifice to the memory of my beloved late Father – Fred Johnson. If it wasn't for him and the love we had for each other I would not be here today. He will always be my hero!

Outline

I.   What Is Wrong With My Baby?

    A. I was a very sick baby when I was born, no one could figure out what was wrong with me.

    B. I was six months old and very near death when a doctor finally diagnosed me with Cystic Fibrosis.

II.   Slow Recovery

    A. My parents had to learn about giving me breathing treatments, postural drainage (to loosen chest congestion), medicines, and take me for numerous doctor visits.

    B. I had to sleep in a mist tent every night in order to keep my lungs clear enough so that I could breathe as I slept.

III. Loving Care

    A. I learned to ignore other peoples remarks about my terrible coughing spells and my discolored teeth.

    B. Each holiday was made very special for me, just in case it was my last.

    C. I missed alot of school because I was sick often; and we had to stay away from other kids when a cold or the flu was going around.

    D. I learned to hold back my coughs when I was around anyone else, to keep track of my medicines and answer questions about Cystic Fibrosis.

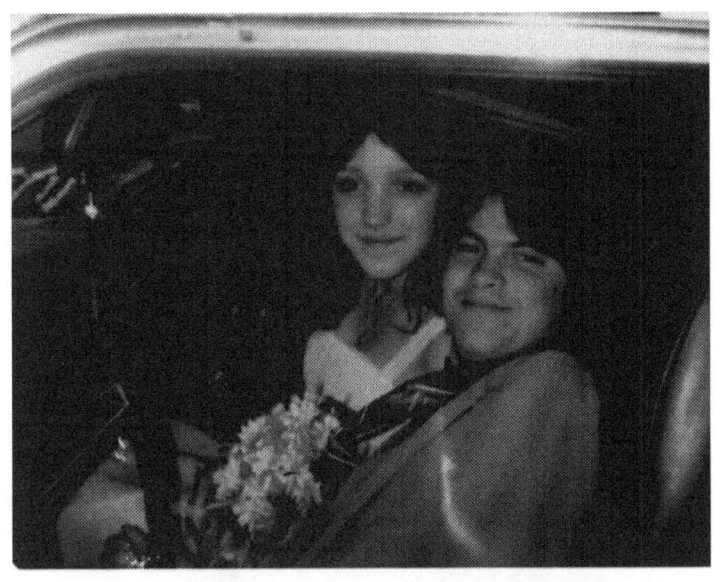

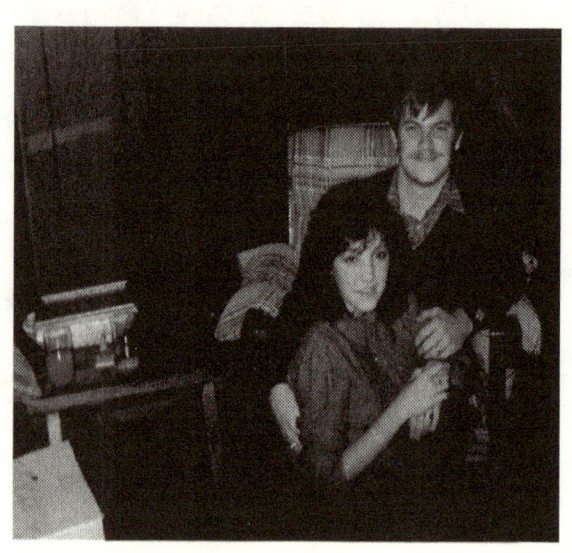

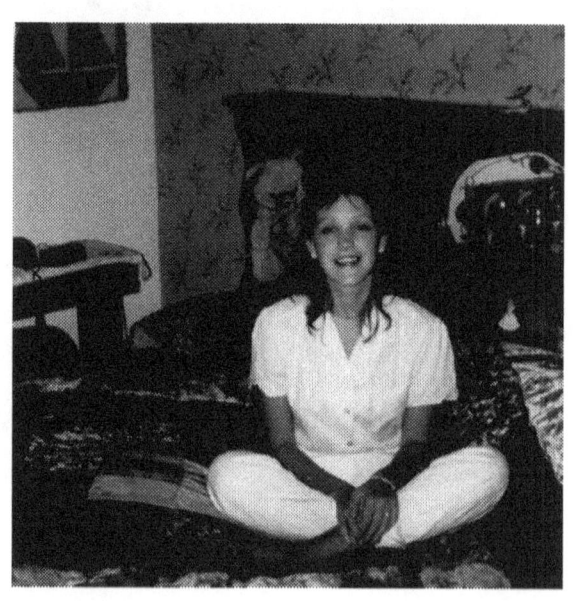

NURSE TACKLES PATIENT WISH

Sometimes taking care of a patient means helping make their wishes come true. Julie Meads, RN, 6A, knew that patient Debbie Pitts of Leesburg was a devoted fan of football star Dan Marino. For months, Meads worked to find a way for Pitts to have a souvenir of her sports idol. Ken Avery, head of Nashville's NFL Alumni, helped make Debbie's wish come true. Avery has a Sout Thomas connection too. His son Jodi works in our OR.

Pictured with Pitts when she received her autographed photo of Dan the Man on Thursday, June 5 were: Avery, husband Jimmy and Meads. Debbie Pitts died Monday, June 9.

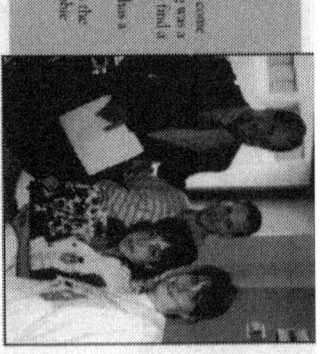

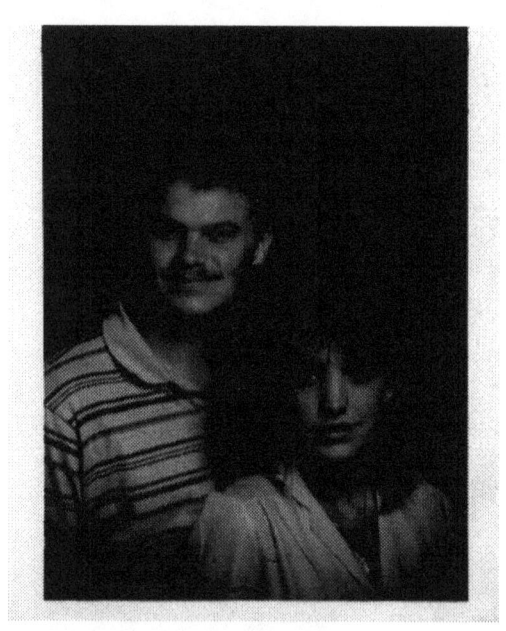

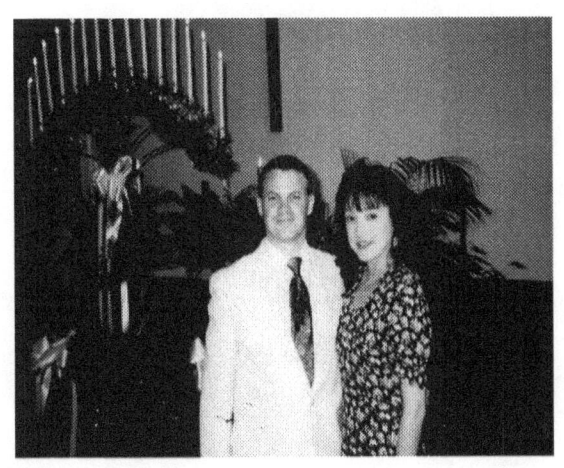

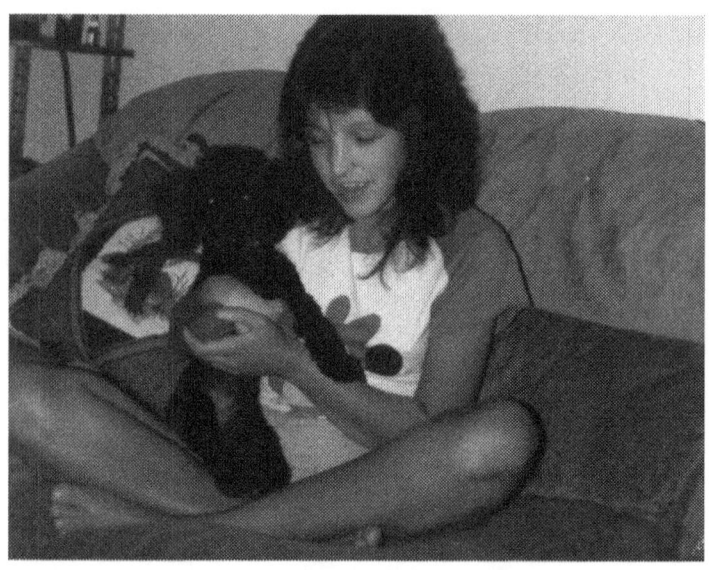

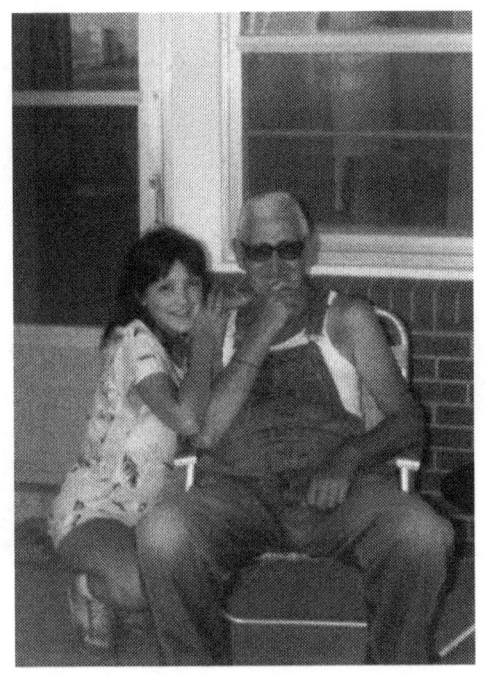

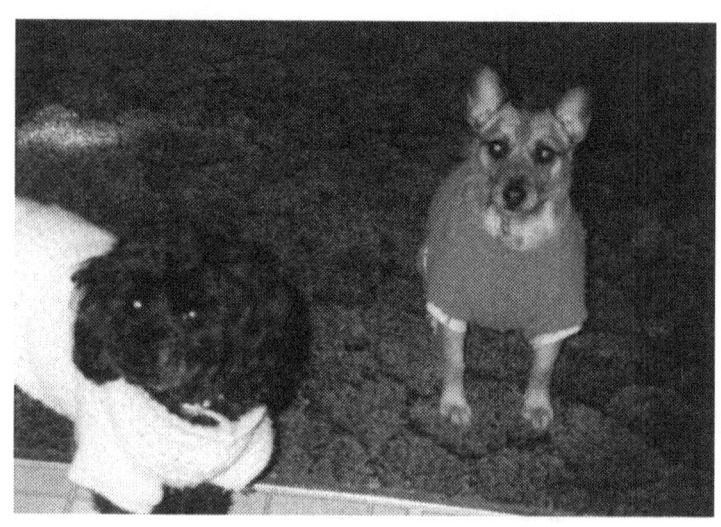

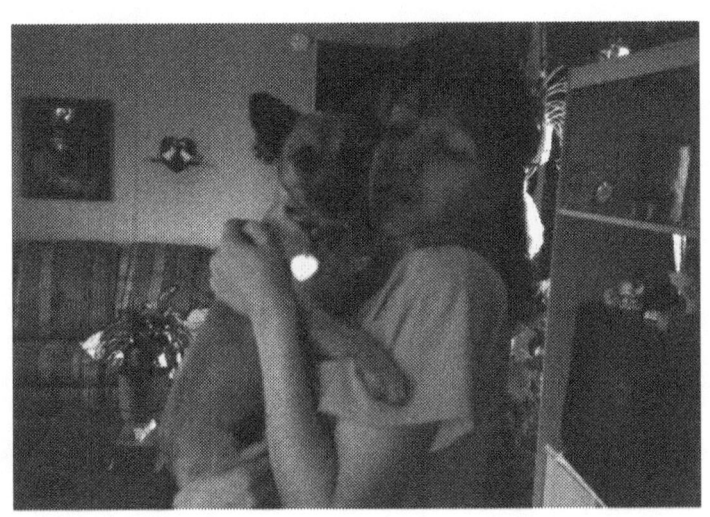

Chapter 1

What Is Wrong With My Baby?

Growing up in Chicago, Illinois during the 60's was a really tough thing for a young family with a new baby born with Cystic Fibrosis. My parents knew right after they took me home from the hospital when I was born that something wasn't quite right with me. I was really small, and sickly. I was not at all like other babies. I was always sick, wheezy, and congested. They took me from one doctor and hospital to another, and no one could figure out what was wrong with me. They were not about to give up on me. My parents fought the cold winter weather and all of my problems with all they had. One day when I was six months old (in December of 61) I was diagnosed at Childrens Memorial Hospital as having Cystic Fibrosis. The main clue that led to my diagnosis was a salty taste on my parents lips after they kissed my forehead.

I was so sick by that time that I was near death and sinking fast. Dr. Rolley vowed to do all he could to save me. He gave my parents a glimmer of hope that I might live for a month, maybe two. He had a big job to do just getting me through one day to the next. Everyone had a big job ahead of them.

The question that kept coming up was how did I end up with CF when no one else in our family has it? I had so many symptoms: salty skin, big appetite but poor weight gain, a chronic cough which produced thick mucus, wheezing, etc...

The reason for me having CF my parents were about to learn. Daddy really tried to learn all he could about this disease; Mom could not handle the details of what to expect.

The doctors described to my parents how the CF gene is carried on down from family members in some families; and it's not always known when two "carriers" of the gene marry. If they have a baby, there is a one in four chance it will have CF. But it will be a carrier. A woman with CF may be able to have children if she is in good enough health. However, the added pressure on her lungs during pregnancy may cause problems. This was what I was later told as I became an adult. I also know that most men with Cystic Fibrosis are not always able to bear children, because they are sterile. Thankfully there are test that can be done to check for the hereditary CF gene.

My daddy had been married before he met my mom. He had a little girl that was very sick. She died when she was about a year or so old. Although it was not proven, we all felt like she may have had CF. Maybe that's why I was so special to my daddy.

My parents learned all about how CF effects the lungs of it's victims. It also makes the digestion of food harder, so special enzymes are needed. Cystic Fibrosis is not a curable disease. It usually causes so many problems that most of the babies born with CF don't live beyond their teen years. The doctors told my parents that I would have numerous lung infections, and probably would need frequent hospital stays. My parents were over-whelmed at what they were hearing. They also felt guilty because I was born so sick. They would learn from trial and error about taking care of a CF baby.

So much had to be done to clear up my pneumonia and get me well. It was going to take several weeks of being in the hospital and getting special care after I was able to go home. The weeks dragged on and on.

CHAPTER 2

Slow Recovery

Slowly I began to respond to all the treatments that the hospital had started. We did not live close to the hospital, so my parents had to use the bus or taxicabs to get me back and forth from home to Childrens Hospital. They learned all about how to do postural drainage (light pounding on my back, sides and chest) to loosen the congested little lungs of their tiny baby.

I was in and out of the hospital for most of the first four years of my life. Each year the doctors would say that I was getting stronger and alot tougher, then they would say that I may just live another year or so. More hope and encouragement was given to my parents. As this happened, they became even more positive that they could help pull me through the hard times; with alot of hope and prayers.

I had a mist tent to sleep in at home. It was a very scary experience for a child to go through, so my bed was in my parents room. Each night I had to crawl into bed and have this big, plastic type of tent pulled down over my bed and tucked into the sides and bottom of the mattress (my own silent, hated, plastic world). Then the switch would be turned on and a cool, foggy mist would start to fill the tent and I would drift off to sleep. My parents always got up to check on me during the night, and helped me when I got choked. My hair was always wet and I looked like I had just gotten out of the shower each morning from the mist tent. I had my tent until I was about six years old. I also had a breathing machine for aerosol treatments that I needed several times during the day and night.

By this time I was in the hospital so much that my parents felt like my own personal doctor and nurse. They could tell by the way I coughed if I was getting sick again. If I sneezed one too many times they knew to call the doctor for certain medicines. Each move I made was watched by them. Especially by my daddy, I was the apple of his eye and his special little girl. Mom would be feeding me when he came home from work, and I would see him and go crazy. I would start yelling and tossing food all over the place; it would end up in my hair, ears, eyes, everywhere! This would not stop until he picked me up and cuddled me.

I guess this was one good way for me to get exercise. This was about the only time I got so carried away. Each day I would end up eating about the same time, waiting for my daddy to come home. It had to be done mainly for the purpose of me getting some exercise.

My brother and sister had to be closely watched too. My parents would make sure that they didn't play with anyone sick or just feeling bad. They had to be careful not to get near me if they had a cold themselves. My brother, Terry, is older; and my sister, Sheila, is younger. They didn't always appreciate not being able to build snowmen or play like normal kids. Coming from Chicago, it was very unusual for kids to stay indoors after a big snow. The whole neighborhood would get out and play in the snow, build snowmen, igloos, and make snowangels. I can remember hearing my parents tell us kids that we could not go out because I might get sick.

Then I would feel bad because I had caused Terry and Sheila to miss out on their fun. Sometimes, though, I would beg Mom and Daddy to let them go out anyway. I would say that I didn't feel like going out, so I would just watch out the window. Then they could go out for a half hour or so. They would be so bundled up that they could hardly move. They would race out and start grabbing up snow. They would always turn towards the window to show me it was for me, and I would stand there with my face up close to the window watching them. I felt so different and sad. But they were having fun and I was glad for them. They would often come back in before they were supposed to; probably because I looked so lonely standing there at the window with my nose pressed against the cold glass.

I can remember these times so well. I also remember a time when Daddy was very sick in the hospital. Mom was home with us kids, and I had been sick. Daddy called to say he was leaving the hospital and coming home. He needed to get back to work, but the doctor would not release him. So he was leaving anyway. I was so glad he was coming home. I told him I wanted a hotdog from one of those street corner vendors. Daddy only had enough money for the bus fare home. It was a ride several city blocks home, or his baby a hotdog. He got my hotdog and walked home with it. I ate it too.

It tears me up to think of this story. I was so young, I didn't realize what I was asking of him. He should have said no, but he didn't. He was still so sick. He just wanted to come home to his family. And since he could not get a work release from his doctor, he had to worry about looking for a new job as well. This man was a true hero to us. We all knew that Daddy would take care of us, no matter what.

CHAPTER 3

Loving Care

It was this kind of special care that kept me out of the hospital too. From the age of four up until I was twenty I was sick alot; but, my parents took care of me at home. Mom was my own private nurse I guess you could say. She'd have to listen to me beg her to skip an aerosol treatment, postural drainage, or a doctors visit. Of course Daddy had to hear me plead too. He'd just say "Do it for me", and I would. Most of the time I was bribed to go to the doctor with a new doll or toy. I had to go to Childrens Hospital every couple of weeks for a check-up and medicine refills.

Each Sunday while most men were busy watching football or relaxing, my daddy was sitting at the kitchen table with a pile of powdered enzymes and a bag of empty, clear capsules. He'd sit there for hours making up enzyme pills to last me until the next weekend. See, the powder was supposed to be mixed in my food, only I had decided long ago that it tasted nasty. I would eat my food that it was mixed in and make faces because it tasted bad. One day Daddy tasted my food and said "No way was I going to be made to eat that". And he started fixing the capsules and taught me to swallow them. I was just a little girl of four or five years, but I learned to take as many pills at one time to get it over with. I later referred to all my pills as my main course of whatever meal I was eating. Then the food was my reward!

I guess that even with all the lung infections, bad colds and hundreds of serious coughing spells (or CF attacks; as I called them) I was better off than most of the other CF children that I was aware of.

The part of being sick that upset me the most was going to the hospital at all times of the day and night. I was scared that they would keep me there and I would never come home again. And when I went for my annual check-ups I would see the same little kids for awhile, then all of a sudden they would disappear. I would ask where they were and I would get a sad look. I knew then that they were in Heaven. I tried not to show how much it scared me then.

I had to toughen up, so I did. My teeth were badly discolored from living off of Tetracyline antibiotics. My fingertips are larger than normal, this is called clubbing. My toes are the same way. The doctor explained that this is caused by a deficiency of oxygen in the bloodstream. Kids at school were cruel, and called me names alot. Names like: rotten teeth or witch fingers. It hurt when they said those things; I thought that I looked pretty normal. Daddy and Mom always said that I looked beautiful. I felt different though. My baby teeth had been pearly white, then my adult teeth had came in a deep, dark brown color because of those antibiotics. It was devastating for me. These days Tetracyline is not usually given to babies in large doses, because of forming teeth.

I became very withdrawn because of these things. I would tell people that I was not the sick girl in our family. I always stayed as close to one of my parents as I could. I was not like other kids and I got tired of trying to be. Why did I have to have CF? No one could give me a good enough answer for that question.

Christmas time and birthdays really were different at our house. I always seemed to get more special gifts, but my parents made sure that each of us kids got more than our share of gifts. They worked very hard to equal out each of the special occasions as they rolled around. Most of the time my daddy worked two jobs so we could have the things that we wanted. We never knew if the holiday we were celebrating would be my last; so each one was made very special.

I came to dread my birthdays. I just knew that it could be my last because I had picked up on the fear that my parents felt. I still feel this way. I always have been quick to pick up on what other people are feeling.

Each time I got sick I could see the pain in my parents eyes. It was always on my mind to try to hide any type of discomfort that I may have been having at the time. In fact; when I was having a bad coughing spell, I always made sure that Mom was the one to help me. Daddy just got so tore up, when those happened that I could not stand for him to see me coughing and choking until I threw up.

When times were hard and everyone else had hamburger on their plates for supper at our house, I had steak on my plate. It was just the way it needed to be since I was so underweight and needed extra proteins and food. I had a big appetite too. My parents were helping me to live, and they did a wonderful job. My brother and sister understood why things were the way they were. They even helped with my treatments, and counting out my medicine at mealtime. We all had to grow up fast in my family. Each member took his or her job seriously. Now you can understand why I felt so out of place, I just wanted to be treated like other kids.

I went to public schools even though it was advised by some doctors that I have a home tutor. We were just very careful about flu season and when colds were going around. Those were the times that I had to stay home. My teachers were always very understanding and helpful.

I always made very good grades, even though I missed alot of school days. In the sixth grade I missed sixty-three days and still passed. I actually got a double-promotion that same year. I worked so much that I would sometimes fall asleep at night with a book in my hand. My daddy would carry me off to bed and tuck me in for the night. And if I woke up I would sometimes start to study again under the covers with a flashlight. I was making sure that I was good at something. Even after getting a double-promotion I faced ridicule from the other students. Some of them would call me "smarty pants" or "the brain". Those names were okay with me. I was used to ignoring people. I was blending in with the other smart kids then, and that was great for me. I was getting special treatment and rewards along with the other kids that got good grades. I finally found a way to fit in and still keep my secret about having Cystic Fibrosis. Only my teachers knew about it.

Mom would bring our lunch to school along with my aerosol pump. We would go off to a secluded room and eat, then I would take aerosol and cough. It was like having a picnic lunch (except for my breathing treatment). Mom did not do the pounding on my back at school, unless I needed some. She would just do a quick version then.

We did not always live close to school so it was quite a trip for Mom to make while carrying a bag of lunch and a heavy breathing machine. She made the trip each day with all that stuff. If it was pretty outside she would meet us at school and walk home with us for lunch and then back to school again. We weren't allowed to walk all that way alone since it was too far.

It did not matter how I got my treatments, I just had to be away from everyone else before I could really cough and clear out my lungs for the rest of the day. I just managed to hold it all in somehow, until the coast was clear for me to cough and not be noticed.

When I was a little girl and had to learn to clear out my lungs I would follow my brother around. He had a habit of spitting just to be doing it. I copied him, until Mom said spitting was not ladylike. So then I had to learn that I should only spit after I coughed and needed to spit. What a job to teach a little kid, it was confusing to me. So we started carrying alot of tissues with us. Then all I had to worry about was finding something to hide behind to use a tissue when I needed to.

It was never possible for me to spend the night at my friends homes when they had slumber parties etc ... I had too much that needed to be done and so many rules that I never did it. I was embarrassed when I coughed hard and I always have to when I wake up each morning; or just turn over during the night after sleeping on one side too long during the night.

When I have one of these coughing fits I get so red in the face, tears stream down my face, and I sound so scary that people look at me like I have some contagious disease. No way was I going to ask to stay with my friends and go through this agony in front of them. Most of my friends just had the impression that CF was sort of like asthma only worse. Wonder how they got that idea?

There have been alot of times when people would ask me what it's like to have Cystic Fibrosis. If I chose to let them even know I have it, that is. I have always had a hard time explaining it. But it's like a regular person having a really bad, congested chest cold. One when it is hard to catch your breath or get air into your lungs. My lungs hurt all the time from coughing and getting my "beatings" as I call them. Only I feel this way each and every day. When I get sick it is much worse, I feel like I am literally going to smother.

My lungs ache continuously. They throb and hurt all of the time. I never get much of a break from it. I just feel bruised and sore from coughing so hard. I try not to complain though. That doesn't help anything. But every once in awhile I have to have a good, long cry and maybe a little self-pity too. Then I'm good for a little longer. A person can only take so much and I figure I have earned the right!

I have approximately ten different medicines that I take on a daily basis. Plus, my aerosol treatments every four hours. I also have two inhalers that I use to help me breathe. Can you imagine having to keep up with all of this? It seems like my entire day is surrounded with what pill is due, and when is my breathing treatment due. If I do want to do anything on a certain day I have to make sure I have all my things with me. It's no fun to do anything this way. It keeps me from doing things even when I feel like it, because I have to pack like I'm going on a trip or something.

CHAPTER 4

We are Moving

Our favorite vacation place was Tennessee. Daddy was born there, and it is a beautiful place. We always hated to go back to the big city of Chicago after a vacation in the country. We all felt better in the clean atmosphere of a small town. We felt so much safer too. So, on one of our vacations Daddy and Mom decided to apply for a job in our favorite vacation spot.

A few weeks later we were making plans to move. And finding a new doctor for me. So much had to be done in a short period of time. My parents were leaving behind alot of things. Mainly, my daddy's career at the factory where he had worked for so long. He was in charge of one of the departments there, and had alot of seniority. He liked his job very much. We also left behind most of my relatives. This was all done in hope of making a better life for our family. No one ever complained of the sacrifices we made.

I was going to start over fresh in a new school, and I had to figure out new ways to cover up my health problems without telling too many people about it. The principal at the new school called me and my parents into the office when we went to register for the eighth grade. He felt like I should go ahead and ignore the double-promotion that I had gotten in Chicago, because of the difference in the school curriculums. He felt that the southern schools were much more difficult to adjust to. My parents assured him that I could do the work and make passing grades in the eighth grade. So a trial basis was set up for me. If I did not meet the standards the principal had set for me within a period of six weeks, I would have to take the seventh grade and give up my promotion.

The heat was on! I had just six weeks to prove what I was made of; and make above average grades in every course. Many of the courses I had were not even similar to my old school subjects from up north. It was difficult to adjust to them, but I did it. And when we all had to meet again the principal was very surprised. Needless to say I got to stay in the eighth grade.

I had more teachers that had to know about my lung problems. Each subject (I had six) had a different teacher. And word got out that I was sick. The questions started to roll in from students. I was stared at and pointed at often. Some kids just wanted to get to know the girl that was "dying". They actually told me that. Can you imagine how I felt hearing that? I was devastated, and wanted to give up on school all together and just stay home. Only after a long talk with my parents, I decided that it really wasn't the kids fault that they had hurt my feelings so badly. I just had to hold my head up high and keep going. I just ignored most of the remarks that were made. My few close friends knew about my having CF; but they never really made a big issue out of it. And finally things settled down with everyone else, and I blended in as usual.

One winter after we had moved to Tennessee we were excited about a light snow that had fallen. It was our second winter here, and it seemed almost tropical compared to the blizzards we had in Illinois. The weather was warm and the light snow looked so pretty on the hills and valleys where we lived. They called school off because of the snow covered backroads, so we had the day to goof off.

Me, my sister and brother begged Mom to let us go out and make snowangels and play in the snow. Mom was not so keen on the idea at first; but she came around and even decided to go out with us. We had so much fun that day. My daddy was at work so he didn't know about the escapade until he got home. At first we thought that maybe we should not bother him with the details of our day. But then we figured that we should go on and tell him, just in case one of us got a cold from our adventure. We were honest to a fault.

We told Daddy that we had all bundled up and went rushing out to play, but we had only been out for a little while. We filled him in on all the fun we had rolling on the snow covered ground, and having snowball fights. It may sound silly to most people, but to me it was magical in a way. I guess Daddy understood how we all felt and he said that it, was okay afterall.

I went on my antibiotics for preventative measures. We did have wood heat in that particular house, so it was extremely warm inside. We felt sort of like pioneers that winter. And I can't remember getting a cold from that time that we all enjoyed our snowday.

Since we lived on a big hill in the country and we wanted to do things like Daddy had done as a child; we tried new things all of the time. Like sleeping on our mattresses by the wood stove. We would drag them in by the woodstove at night and "campout." Mom and Daddy would sit around and tell us their childhood stories. We felt like the Walton family from the television show; plus, we learned so much about our parents and ancestors this way. We even said goodnight to each other every single night individually. Those were the good old days!

Living on that big hill was an experience I'll never forget. Our driveway was approximately half a mile long. One good rain, and we would be knee deep in mudd. It was a slippery mess during the rainy months. We parked at the bottom of the driveway and walked up to the house. We would have to drive down that slippery hill if it rained during the night and hope that we wouldn't get stuck in the mudd. Or even slide off in a ditch! We would be singing and acting like idiots while Mom was easing the car down the road on our way to school, so we would not have to wait in the bad weather for the schoolbus. It's a wonder she didn't lose her mind.

All this was our reasons for moving to the south. Not the bad parts of course, but to live as fulfilled lives as we could and to learn about surviving in different ways. In Chicago, we could not go out of the yard without fear of the unknown. Living here in a small town we felt safer and almost like we had been set free. We loved it. And it felt great!

I did miss alot of high school, as usual. I had to work harder than ever to keep up a B+ average. Most subjects I had A's in though. My favorite subjects were literature and office education. Mrs. Shirley Coates was my office education teacher. She really is a wonderful lady, I see her often. Mrs. Coates always seemed to pay special attention to my needs without drawing attention to me. If I had a bad spell with coughing I could just give her a look and leave the room without special permission. She'd ask if I was okay when I came back in (sometimes it was 5 or 10 minutes later before I came back). I always enjoyed going to her class. It was her encouragement and guidance that made me do so well in her class. I competed in several competitions having to do with office work, and I won several first and second place ribbons. I was even listed in the Who's Who Among American High School Students book because of Mrs. Coates class. I had quite a few favorite teachers during high school, they all made a big impact on my way of thinking and the way I learned to deal with my special problems. I hope they all know how special they are to me.

CHAPTER 5

The Task Of A New Job

One day I decided I wanted to get a job after school. My friend said there was an opening where she worked at the local hangout. It was an ice cream place. She knew she could help get me the job if I wanted it. I begged my parents to let me try it. I applied for the position and got it. I was so happy and it was great fun. Seeing all the kids from school coming in and out all the time helped me make new friends.

The jukebox was always playing, and people were always dropping in to say hello. I started to come out of my shell that I had always lived in little by little. And then about two weeks later another opening came up for night manager. My mom got that position, so we worked after school together. Eventually my sister got a job there too, and it seemed like a family business. People always asked us if we had bought the place. Daddy always stayed close by while we worked our evening and weekend shifts. He helped cook hamburgers and fries. He was always singing along with the the jukebox as he filled the grill orders. Everyone thought that I had the coolest parents they had ever met. Some of the older girls would ask my mom advice about boy problems. It was really the type of place that alot of people would feel comfortable just coming in to sit and talk.

At times I would have to sneak out behind the building to cough so that no one could hear me or see me. Then I would calmly walk back in and go back to work as if nothing had happened. I even took my aerosol pump in the back of the place so I could use it when I needed it. All of this was under the watchful eyes of my family. They could not let me fail at a job that meant so much to me; so they got a job there to help me cover up any problems that might come up.

I guess we had all worked there a couple of years (or close to it) before our boss found out that I was sick. By then he did not care, because we had it under control. I managed to work like this for about three years or so. It was very difficult and I stayed so tired. I could never had kept that job it if wasn't for the help of my family.

I can remember many times when I was too sick to work. I would go in to work with my mom and sister, the boss would leave, and we would all switch places. Daddy would work the grill, mom would take my place at the register, Sheila would do Mom's counter work. Our boss never seemed to mind. He was just happy to have the place in good hands, and have everything taken care of and kept clean. We always made sure that the place was spotless, and the things that were supposed to be filled up was always full.

While all of this was going on I would be in the back room laying my head over on the shelf beside the boxes of straws, cups, and other supplies. Resting on a pile of our jackets. I was too tired to work and too mad at myself to quit working. Finally the place was sold and eventually closed down. What a relief that was, I could rest and say I didn't quit afterall. That was three of the longest, hardest years of my life. Again, the closeness of my family shown like a diamond in the sunlight! I never really carried my share of the load during those years.

All during this time I was working hard at my school work and getting ready for graduation. I was floating on air and full of anticipation. None of us dreamed that I would even live to graduate from anything; let alone high school. I had mixed emotions about graduation. I really did love school and I was going to miss it. Going to college was a dream of mine, but I knew I was not able to go back and forth to an out of town school. And living on a school campus was out of the question for me. So I was just glad that I had made it as far as I had. I was used to making sacrifices anyway. Besides, I could always take a night course at the high school when they offered them. Right now I had a major event to prepare for and I wasn't going to miss a minute of this glory.

During graduation practice I counted out the rows of seats that were placed next to the seats for the seniors. I knew they were for the immediate family members, and I wanted my family to sit right along side of my row. I was the second senior from the end of my row (great luck)! So I told my parents to head for the specific row that would put them just a couple feet away from my seat. It would be like we were all sitting together for this event.

That warm, beautiful evening of June 1, 1979 I walked up to the stage when my name was called, got my diploma, and slowly made my way back to my seat. Pausing for a moment to focus on my family and the tears in their eyes. This was one of the happiest times in my life. After the ceremony was over we went home to celebrate with cake and icecream. The other seniors went to a big party, I could have gone to it, but I wanted to share this time with the people I loved so much. Afterall, they had fought this battle with me.

CHAPTER 6

Jimmy

One night I was lucky enough to meet a very sweet and adorable guy. He had a way about him that just made everyone who knew him like him. His bright blue eyes, and warm smile melted my heart. He was the most polite guy I had ever met. His name was Jimmy. His laughter was almost contagious. There was just something about him that made me feel so happy. Little did I know, but we were soon to fall head over heals in love.

You know how everyone always says that you usually find love when you are not necessarily looking for it? And thats when you meet that "right" person you will just know somehow? Well, that is exactly what happened to us. Out of the blue came this wonderful, loving guy that seemed to be made just for me. He was very concerned about my lung problems, but he didn't run from them.

Soon after our first meeting he called to ask me out on a date. We saw a meteor shower that night in the sky. At first we thought that we had saw a falling star, so we made a wish. Then we saw several more of them and we knew that this was a really unusual date. Later as we were getting ready to go back to my house; we drove past this one store that had a beautiful, long ivory dress hanging in the window. I said something about how pretty it was. Jimmy said that he would buy it for me so we could get married. This was all on our first date! I thought to myself " Either this guy is crazy or just too good to be true". Maybe he was just joking, but he sounded so serious. We never talked about the dress again.

We were rarely ever apart after that first date. Jimmy was a senior in high school, so I called him each morning to make sure that he was up on time and so we could talk a few minutes before he left for school. He later came over to my house before he went to his job that he had weeknights. I always had him a big supper packed to take with him each night. I would fry up a chicken breast, send bread to go with it, and usually some type of cake for desert. I always wrote him a love note and put in the bag too. I had never felt so domesticated before. I made sure that he had a variety of meals so he wouldn't get bored or think that I could only make one type of meal.

We started dating on December 13, 1980; and Jimmy asked me to marry him right before Valentine's Day 1981. A little over two months after we had started dating. We were so much in love, and I immediately said yes. We set the date for the following Valentine's Day, thinking a year would give us time to get things in order. He was so close to graduating from high school, and we had so much to do. Jimmy already had his own place, and he had a job too. He was just so mature for a guy just eighteen years old.

After we had gotten engaged my parents talked to Jimmy and explained to him all about Cystic Fibrosis, and what could happen to me. Jimmy said that he loved me and he wanted to marry me anyway. The fact that he is a year younger than I am was no factor either. We were crazy over each other and we wanted to be together. If anything, the talk with my parents made Jimmy want to move up our wedding date. We wanted to spend every second together that we possibly could.

When we had gotten engaged, Mom had remembered that she had a set of wedding rings that Daddy had given her a long time ago. Since then she had gotten new ones. But I had always loved the older ones that were set in both yellow and white gold. She promised me when I was a little girl that I could have them when I found my "lucky man" and got engaged. I had forgotten about the set of rings over the years.

One day after Jimmy had proposed to me, he pulled out this little ring box and opened it up. There were the set of rings that I had loved for so long. He put the engagement ring on my finger and we left the matching band in the box. We decided to get our own set of matching gold wedding bands the next weekend. As for the one that went with my engagement ring, we would just keep it in the box. The bands we chose for ourselves were beautiful, medium width, gold bands. My ring went perfect with the band we chose. We were elated!

Everyone that knew us said that we were just meant to be together. There seemed to be happiness that floated all around us during those days. People who barely knew us as a couple noticed the magic. We decided to move our wedding day up to the following month. We could not wait to be married, and everything was already set (except for the wedding details) so we said "Let's do it"!

We got married out of town by Jimmy's grandfather. He is a minister at a big beautiful church close to the Tennessee and Arkansas state line. My family could not go since they managed a firehall that had to have someone there at all times to answer the hotline phone. They could not find anyone to stay there the couple of days needed to travel to our wedding, on such short notice. Even alot of Jimmy's family was not there. That has to be the only regret I have about getting married so quickly; my Daddy couldn't give me away and so many of our family members were not there.

Jimmy walked me down the aisle, he kissed me on the cheek and told me that I looked beautiful. I was wearing the very same dress that we had seen in the store window on our first date. He did not know that I had chosen it for our special day. It turned out to be a wonderful day for both of us. We were so happy, we were in love and on top of the world. I'm sure most married couples feel the same way we did on their wedding day; but I never thought I would find such a great guy that would accept me and all of my problems. When Jimmy said "for better or worse" during our ceremony he really meant it.

While we were gone off to be married my family was rushing around to surprise us. They had our refrigerator packed with everything you could imagine. Mom even made a cherry cheesecake (we love those) and put a note beside it on the top shelf of the fridge.

On the kitchen counter were several bags of groceries; packed full of all of my favorite things. They left them on the counter in bags so we could see what we had as we "unloaded" the goodies to put them away.

Over in the middle of the kitchen was a beautiful dinette set that Daddy had bought for us. We had been using a card table and folding chairs when we set the house up for Jimmy to move into. Daddy was afraid that we might not like the table and chairs, since we had not picked it out ourselves. But we loved it. And it was perfect for us.

Before we had left for our wedding we had given my parents a set of keys to the house so they could move in a few last boxes of mine, and to check on things. We had no idea that they had all of the surprises they did for us in mind.

Jimmy had already mastered the art of doing the laundry. He was so smart and seemed to know just how to do everything. All he had to do was to teach me! I could cook, clean, and do most things; laundry was not one of my finer points. I just packed everything in one machine and felt good about it. I finally got the hang of it after awhile, but we still did the laundry and everything else together.

Jimmy has such a large family that it took time for us to make the rounds and get introduced. I was scared that they might not like me, or that they would worry about me having CF. But each and every family member that I met, was absolutely the sweetest and most polite person. They all welcomed me with opened arms. Almost as if they had known me all of my life. That's just the kind of people they are. I could not have asked for a better family to marry into. I really do love them all very much. And since I'm from an open, affectionate kind of family; I make sure to tell them that I love and appreciate them often.

Up until now I had been doing pretty good at keeping down lung infections etc... Of course I had my parents to watch after me. So in general I was feeling good, and only having my normal amount of CF coughing attacks. I was well informed about what I could and could not do. The pollen and ragweeds in this area really make me sick, so I knew to stay in our house of these high pollen count times. Spring was here so, I was on my guard.

Also, Jimmy was getting ready for his graduation from high school. Everything was moving so fast that we could hardly keep up. And then the big day was upon us, and Jimmy was walking down the aisle in his cap and gown for graduation. He had started going to school for only half of the day before we got married because there were not enough hours in a day for all he had to do. We weren't sure if he would get to walk down the aisle with the rest of his class because of this fact. But he was allowed to. I guess he was the only graduating male senior that was married in his class. We were so proud of him. My sister was in the same class; so we were really one big, happy group that night.

CHAPTER 7

Coming Out Of Remission

After Jimmy graduated we moved to Nashville, TN. I had taught him all about doing postural drainage and percussion. We used to joke around and say he got to beat on me; only because I called my treatments "beatings". To me they were like a form of torture because I hate having them. I tried to get by without them as much as I can because I stay so sore from being pounded on. If it isn't done just right it really can hurt a person. So a special way of doing it is taught to parents of CF children.

Even though I was extremely careful, I got the shock of my life one night. Nearly six months to the day after we got married, I was being rushed to the emergency room. I had woke up around midnight with a throbbing ache in my chest. I started to cough and when I spit in the sink it was pure blood. I was having trouble breathing, and my chest was hurting so bad that I started to cry. I screamed for Jimmy, and he came running into the bathroom. I was standing there just spitting blood and crying. Neither of us knew what to do, so we called my doctor and he said to get me to the emergency room fast. He also said I needed to keep calm and realize that this was just part of having CF. That was all news to me since I was always shielded from any information about CF. Before we left the apartment we called my parents to tell them about what was happening. They were upset, but not totally surprised. They were aware of this problem occuring in most CF patients at some point. I wish they had told us about it before it happened to me.

I spent the night in the emergency room for observation. They gave me codeine to suppress my cough. The doctor on duty said I had to remain very still so that the spot that was bleeding could clot off. They took several x-rays off and on during the night. Finally, they let me rest and told me to try to get some sleep. I was too scared to do anything but cry. Jimmy was sitting beside the bed in a hard, plastic chair. He was holding my hand and promised to watch me if I drifted off to sleep. I was afraid I would start to bleed again; or worse, not wake up at all.

That was a really long night for us. Everytime I woke up and looked over at Jimmy, he was awake watching me. He finally lay his head over next to mine and we went to sleep. We slept like that until the nurse came in with more medicine for me and to say we could go home.

Each of us was equally terrified at what we had went through. When we got home we tried to sleep, but we were so scared to do much of anything. Afraid that something would happen if I coughed again, or if I moved to fast. It was a scarey thing. I had this gurgling sound in my throat that night before when I had first started to bleed, so we kept listening for that awful sound again. Jimmy took the day off of work and we just sat around like two scared mice.

I really wanted to be close to my family during this time so, we went home for a visit the next day. Soon after all of this happened we decided to move back home. I was so relieved. I was twenty and Jimmy had just turned nineteen. It all seemed so unfair to us that this could start to be the beginning of our problems. We were newlyweds, and had so much to look forward to. Or should I say, we should have so much to live for and look forward to; now we did not know what was happening to me. Our new life had been so much fun until now.

Ater we first moved to Nashville, we went to movies, swimming at the apartment complex where we lived, the malls shopping, always on the go. Jimmy worked at the complex where we lived and I always followed him around. Sometimes helping him or just watching him work. We were always together. I was missing my family and I needed to be close to Jimmy. I had not made any real friends, so I was lonesome.

Now that we had moved back to the small town where my family lived, we were sort of lost for things to do again. At least we were close to our friends again. And anything we needed we usually went out of town for, so we were not totally lost. At least my family was very close. That made us feel more comfortable about my being sick so much; all we had to do was call them and within minutes they would be there for me. It worked out great.

My, bleeding spells were coming more often, usually at night for some reason. I would wake up with that familiar gurgling sound, and awful ache in my chest. After one cough

I knew it was happening again. I would move towards the bathroom and brace myself for however long it took to calm the bleeding down. Jimmy would get me a codeine, a cool washcloth, and hold me over the sink while I coughed. I usually wheeze really bad at these times too. After a few minutes of panic I would go back to bed, prop up on a stack of pillows with an icepack on my chest and lean against my main source of support, Jimmy. There is always a box of tissue and a small basket for trash beside my bed.

I was covered by a program called Crippled Childrens Service (or CCS) until I turned twenty-one. My medical bills were covered, as long as I went to a certain hospital in Nashville. And I was nearing my twenty-first birthday.

From the time of my first bleeding spell in the fall of 1981, I was in and out of the hospital. Two days after our first Christmas as a newlyweds, I was being rushed by ambulance to the hospital in Nashville. I had a bad case of pneumonia and I could not stop bleeding. Jimmy rode with me, while my parents drove over the speed limit behind the ambulance. This was all getting to be too much for me to cope with. I was scared to death! Not to mention the fear my family and friends were living with. After I was settled in the hospital bed, my parents reluctantly went home. They returned the next morning with everything I needed, and some things for Jimmy as well. He had refused to leave my side.

I was released from the hospital after several days. I had to promise to go home and stay in bed for several days. Only getting up to go to the bathroom. Luckily, my daddy had gone over to our house to clean up the blood that had splattered all over the bathroom while I was throwing up, before I had went into the hospital. Mom and Sheila had tried to clean up the mess, but they got sick when they saw all the blood. Daddy said it looked like someone had been killed in that place. I had tried to aim for the toilet or the sink when I had gotten sick; but blood splatters so much. I was also getting sick all throughout the house, and could not hold it back.

Thank goodness our place was spotless when we got home. I could not have taken any more reminders of that awful experience. What a way to start off a new year.

I gave up on the CF doctor that I was seeing. We just did not have a good patient and doctor relationship. In fact I rarely seen him; usually I saw a different intern that knew nothing of my specific condition. It was like seeing a new doctor every time I went for a visit. I wanted and needed a one on one situation with a caring doctor. I needed help fast and I needed a good doctor I could count on. We were not covered by CCS; since I had turned twenty-one, so I had no insurance.

We decided to try Dr. Collins at the clinic in the next town. We explained the situation to him and asked for his help. He is not a CF specialist, but he said he knew alot about CF. He said he would like to help me and he would be willing to learn all he could about Cystic Fibrosis. I had found a doctor that really cared about his patients. Dr. Collins is a very nice person. I felt like I had found a doctor that I could count on; and I had.

CHAPTER 8

Why Me?

The months went by slowly and I started to feel better. Jimmy and I were trying to put our lives back on track. During late summer in 1983, it was so hot. I had been sick and having trouble with all of my allergies. Then a summer cold came on; I was feeling congested alot more. I was needing my aerosol and "beatings" more often, they could not seem to clear my lungs out. Then I started running a high fever. Something was wrong and we put off going to the doctor, because I kept thinking I would get better. Plus we still had no insurance for me yet.

One night I woke up bleeding really bad. We were used to it by now, but this time it was different. We couldn't get it to stop. We got in the car and rushed to the hospital. Dr. Collins was called and had me admitted immediately. The hospital was not so happy with my not having insurance. Dr. Collins talked to the office personnel and they took care of my bill.

After being on oxygen and large doses of antibiotics for several days, I thought I was getting a little better. Mom, Sheila, and some of Jimmy's friends were all visiting me one night. I was tired and dozing off and on while they were chatting away. All of a sudden I began to cough hard. The bleeding started again with a vengeance. The nurses began running all around calling for help. They told everyone in the room to leave; and they started working on me fast. I'll never forget the way they held that oblong dish up for me to throw up in. I'm talking about the dish they gave me when I checked into the hospital. I filled it full of pure blood, and then they grabbed the larger plastic pan that looked like a dishpan. I filled it over half full of blood.

Nothing was stopping this maddness. By this time everyone was hysterical. Some of the nurses were in the hall with my family, and all of them were crying (nurses, too). My family was advised to get the rest of my family there. Daddy was home, and Jimmy was at work. They came rushing in within a few minutes. Then a little later on Jimmy's dad came in from Nashville. My doctor arrived about the same time as Jimmy had, and told everyone I was critical. They were not sure I would live through the night.

They began giving me morphine to help me calm down. They told me to get some sleep and that I had to be very still so the bleeding could stop. I was too scared to sleep and I fought the sleepy feeling from the drug with all I had in me. They gave me another large syringe full of morphine. Enough they said would knock a grown man out. I still tried to stay awake. I just knew I would never wake up if I went to sleep. My chest was hurting so bad, and I had gotten blood all over my pretty new nightgown that Mom had gotten me. I was told that my gown was not important and my resting was. Daddy held my hand and said he'd watch me while I slept. So I finally said I would get some rest.

A little while later Dr. Collins came in again, and he said he wanted to send me to a Nashville hospital that was more "up" on taking care of this type of situation. I was asked what I wanted to do. I said I did not want to go anywhere else. That I had all the faith in the world in Dr. Collins, and I wanted to be close to my family. I also said that if I was going to die I wanted to do it with all the people that I love around me.

Daddy never left my bedside that night. Everytime I woke up, he and Mom were there. I could here them crying and begging God to let me live. I could feel Daddy rubbing my left hand so softly all that night. Jimmy was there all night too, but later he went to get some rest in the waiting room with all of the family members. I was worried that Jimmy needed rest because he had been several hours without any sleep. So everyone promised that they would rest so that I would rest. It was a very long night.

Mom and Sheila took turns staying the nights with me. Jimmy was always there and he stayed nights with me, too. Daddy was with me every second that he had free. I was so weak and sick that I needed around the clock care; my family gave me that care, along with the nurses. That way I didn't have to go into the critical care unit. They only allow short, immediate family visits, every few hours. I had so many people wanting to be with me, that being in that unit would have been hard on me and my family. We all needed to be as close to each other as we could.

My blood pressure was extremely low and I was turning a blue color (my lips were almost purple). They checked my blood level and said I was dangerously low. I would need blood transfusions fast. They gave me four bags of whole blood. It made me nauseated to see that blood running in my arm, so they covered the bags with a towel to hide them.

The nurses were checking my vital signs every fifteen minutes to make sure there were no problems. But I was still so weak and sick that I could not raise my head. Looking back now, I can't understand where my strength came from to fight that terrible time and still live. I must have drawn energy from all the people that surrounded me with love, prayers, and of course the excellent medical care I received. Dr. Collins even called the doctors that had first diagnosed me as having CF when we lived up north. They still remembered me after all those years as being a fighter.

In the meantime, cards and get well wishes came pouring in from people I did not even know. Mom would tape them to the window so I could see them. There were at least fifty of them. I also got flowers and stuffed animals from everywhere. Even the nurses came to see me on their days off. Some of them brought me gifts to cheer me up. It was a long uphill battle; but, after a little over two weeks I got to go home. I was hesitant to go home, I must admit. I was so scared that something would happen and I would bleed to death or something.

Dr. Collins said I had to promise to stay in bed for a while and not do anything. My family would have to help me. People were taking turns bringing our supper to us each day. And someone was usually with me while Jimmy was at work.

It took at least six months for me to fully recover. I have never been the same since. I was fighting to get on disability during this time. It is never easy to get that, so I was staying upset alot, when I should have been resting. I had to go through so much just to prove I was sick that I started having problems again. Dr. Collins could not understand why I was having such a hard time proving that I was disabeled. He helped me all he could. And I had to go on nerve pills just to keep me calm. It got to where I could not sleep, eat, or do much of anything because of worrying. Finally, I got my disability so I had some insurance now. I'm not sure which was worse; getting well or getting on disability. Dealing with both subjects really drained me of what little energy I had left. I remember thinking that I might be able to sit back and rest now.

CHAPTER 9

A New Change

A year or so later we tried moving back to Nashville. There just wasn't much work available in that small town we were living in. We thought we would give Nashville another try. I was still having some bad spells, but by now we felt like pro's at handling them. I always had my different medicines for different problems close at hand; codeine, pain medicine, and nerve pills. After awhile I just knew what to take when certain problems would crop up. I also knew that I had to stay calm or else it just made matters worse.

After all the things we have gone through; I found myself becoming obessed with being with Jimmy. More than I had ever been before. I even started to have panic attacks when he was not around. Whenever we would go someplace I have to be right beside him. If some other family member or close friend is there instead, I'm the same way. But, I'm more prone to my panic spells with Jimmy. If I look around and cannot find a familiar face, I panic. I start to sweat and get scared. It's hard for me to hold back tears at times. Sometimes I just stand in one spot and watch for him, or I have searched frantically until I find him. It's a very upsetting thing to happen to a person. I usually don't go anywhere alone if I can help it. I have went into a store with a list of things to get, and had to leave without any of the things because I had a panic attack. For a long time I never told anyone about this, it was embarrassing to me. Now, it's just a fact of life with me.

I cannot imagine my life without Jimmy. He is my absolute best friend. I love him more than I could ever express in words. We know what each other is thinking most of the time. Jimmy is a very strong, good man for standing beside me with all of my problems. I'm not so sure that many people would be able to deal with all we have to deal with.

I belong to Jimmy, heart and soul for the rest of my life. He spoils me, and I try to spoil him as much as I can. Our life is very difficult; we lean on each other for support and love. We just wish we that our lives could be more normal. I would give anything to be normal. To have a regular job, a boring life, would be great. As long as we could just have our good health, I would never complain. It really makes me mad to see people laying around doing nothing with their lives. When they are capable of doing so much. Alot of people just sit back and ask for things (and they usually get it). I just cannot tolerate that kind of behavior. I hate wanting to do simple things so bad and not being able to do them. I get out of breath just walking across the room; or taking a shower even exhausts me.

As crazy as it sounds I wanted to try to work again after we moved back to Nashville. I was starting to feel so worthless and depressed. My self-esteem was really low. I begged Jimmy to let me try to work. To prove to myself if I could do it or not.

I stayed tired most of the time, but my bad bleeding spells were further apart now. Everyone said I should just accept things as they were and not consider a job. I had other plans though.

About a month or two after being back in Nashville; Jimmy's step-mother (Donna) offered me a job at the apartment complex where we lived. She was the manager there. I was so thrilled! I said I wanted the job right away, and I took it. Dr. Collins was very against it. Jimmy was not so happy about it, but he said I could try it for awhile. He knew it meant so much to me. My family was worried; but, they also knew it meant alot to me. I promised everyone I that I would be very careful and quit if it got too difficult. I really did mean it when I made that promise; but, I loved my job so much. I guess I pushed myself too far.

My job was so great. Donna was extra watchful over me. She was always letting things slip by that other workers might not get by with. Like when I had a bad spell, I got to go home. If I woke up sick I just called in, or if I was needing an extra aerosol treatment; I just went up to our apartment and took it. Then I would go back to work if I was feeling better. I did miss several days. Having my mother-in-law for a boss was an added benefit for me. She helped me out in alot of ways. I'll always be grateful to her for giving me a chance to prove something to myself.

I have to admit, though, she did seem pleased with my work. And I did work hard to please her. I didn't want to let her down. I did office work at my desk, collected rent, dealt with new tenants, wrote leases etc... It was the perfect job for me. Working and talking to people made me feel important. I loved it.

I worked with another girl, Sandy, who turned out to be a very good friend to me. She would show apartments on my bad days, or if the weather was bad. Even Donna did the same thing for me. They were always worried that I would catch a cold or wear myself out. They covered for me so well. I always appreciated their help. We all helped each other out. Sandy and I alternated working on weekends. We were both considered assistant managers. I was twenty-three now and I really felt important. I hid the fact that I was starting to feel exhausted after only a couple of months of working. I would work eight hours each day (sometimes less), go home and eat some supper, then go to sleep on the sofa. I would not be able to stay awake past 8 o'clock most nights. I was getting run down, but I tried to hide it so hard. I needed to feel important and this job did that for me.

One weekend that I was off, Jimmy and I was riding our motorcycle. Donna and Jimmy's dad, Lynn, were on their own motorcycle in front of us. It was a beautiful day, we were all enjoying ourselves. Then all of a sudden a young guy ran a stop sign, and hit Donna and Lynn. It was like slow motion. They were sliding down the highway head over heels. We were screaming so loud. Terrified that they were hurt bad. It was the most horrifying experience you could imagine. It turned out that they were badly scratched up, bruised, and very sore for quite awhile. That ended our motorcycle days right then.

When you see people that you dearly love nearly killed before your eyes, things take on a new prospective. We sold our bike soon after that. It took a few weeks for things to get back to normal at work; so I didn't say anything about being so tired and thinking about having to give up my job. Donna needed my help in the office, and I was going to help her all that I could.

It was Spring outside and everything was budding out all over. My allergies were really acting up. I had started to bleed again. I was having to go back and forth to see Dr. Collins more often. He would tell me that I needed to stop working. But I was not ready to give up yet. It was a stupid thing to do, I know. By the end of eight months of trying to work, and getting so much help from my co-workers, I was back in the emergency room. I knew this time it was the end of my working career. Dr. Collins said I had to stop working for good this time.

I was so upset about having to quit work. I was doing damage to my lungs each time that I got sick. Damage that could not be reversed. I was exhausted anyway, and I knew it was time to throw in the towel. So that's just what I did.

I actually had been showing an apartment to a couple when I got sick before I ended up in the hospital. I coughed and heard that familiar gurgling in my throat. I just excused myself, went into the bathroom; there it was, blood. I told the people that I had to go to the office to check on something and they should just look around. I sent Donna up to finish showing the apartment. Then I went up to our apartment and got into bed. I waited for Jimmy to come home and take me to the hospital. That's when I really knew it was over for my working days. I was in the hospital for a week, but it felt like alot longer. I was very depressed to say the least.

We continued to live in Nashville for a couple of years after that. We were always having trouble with my insurance coverage. It was difficult to get help and still be a married person. Each penny that Jimmy earned counted against us. He was barely making enough money to pay the bills on his own. We were having to take out loans to buy my medicines and to pay on other loans. We were in debt and not getting any help. Even though I was sick and needed it.

We were trying very hard to get by on our own. It was like we were just always running into brick walls. After awhile we were too aggrivated and tired to go on. We had to keep fighting for help, and keep borrowing money. My doctor bills and medicines had to be paid for; and we did the best we could to pay on them a little at a time. It put a big strain on our marriage. We had begun to argue more often.

Chapter 10

A New Doctor And Hospital

By the end of 1986, I had began to see a wonderful lung specialist named Dr. Brevard Haynes. His office in the Saint Thomas Hospital medical building was much closer to our home. I was having so many more problems that I needed a doctor that was close by.

I started breaking Dr. Haynes in right away. He always seemed to know just what to do for me. I was very impressed with him. He realized right off that Jimmy and I were very knowledgeable about my condition (and how to deal with my specific special problems as they came along), more than most people might be. With Cystic Fibrosis, as well as any other serious illness, a person has to have a positive outlook and attitude in order to deal with the everyday stress and life in general.

As one respiratory therapist, Pat, said to me; life handed me a bunch of lemons and I just made lemonade with them instead of giving up. Pat works at Saint Thomas Hospital.

She has been one of the therapist that always cheers me up. Whenever I go into the hospital for a "tune up" I manage to see or ask about at least ten of the respiratory people that I know really well. There are always several new ones that I make friends with each time I go in the hospital. My friends that have given me my treatments over the years are very special to me.

My treatments take so long and I get them so often; yet the technicians don't get rushed or impatient with me. They usually have an entire page of patients to see besides me, so they are always busy. If I need an extra treatment they tell me to just call for them. They are the best people.

I consider several of the technicians very dear friends of mine. We catch up on the latest about my dogs and our families. It means alot that they care so much. They even remember my dogs by name, and they always get to see my latest picture of them. Most of them ask about my "special babies" before anything else. They know my dogs mean the world to me.

And I learn from the technicians as I get my long treatments. If I want to learn about a blood gas result, or how my lungs are actually helped by aerosol treatments, or any question I may have about Cystic Fibrosis, I just ask them. Several of the workers have dealt with CF patients in the past. I have questions about CF that I am hesitant to ask some people. I know that I can ask one of them for the answer and they will tell me. They get me through some sad and lonely times. I hope Saint Thomas Hospital and their respiratory department know just how lucky they are to have so many caring people working for them.

The Fall and Winter of 1986, was a very sick time for me. I was in and out of Saint Thomas every couple of months. Before long I came to know so many of the people there; from nurses, I.V. therapists, food servers, to cleaning people., Whenever I got checked in they would start rolling in to say hello. And to make sure that I was doing okay or needing anything. They are like a second family to me.

Since my family lived over an hour away, Jimmy was the only visitor I ever had. The long drive was hard for Daddy to make so he called me everyday. Mom said she could not drive in Nashville's traffic. So each time I went in the hospital I was very depressed. I tried not to let people see it though. I always felt like the nurses and therapist could use a smile and I would try to give them one, no matter how bad I felt.

Sleeping in the hospital is one thing I cannot do. I'm usually awake whenever someone would come into my room for whatever reason. One night in particular I was getting my breathing treatment and "beating", when the respiratory guy started to raise the bed up to position it for my beating. To do that they have to raise the bed up high, tilt the head down, then lower the bed to the height they need it to be. So they can reach me comfortably to pound on my back. Then they would put the bed back in the regular position and I was done until the next time. This one night the guy doing my treatment started to raise the bed and something popped when he went to stop it from going up. I was stuck up above five feet or more in the air. We didn't know what to do. He started calling for the nurse and maintenance worker. All I could see were the tops of their heads. It was weird. Everyone wanted to be sure that I stayed calm. They did all they could to get the bed to lower, it would not budge.

The therapist was getting upset, thinking he had done something wrong. It wasn't his fault. I couldn't hold back any longer. I started to laugh. Here it was about 2 o'clock in the morning and I'm stuck up in the air in my hospital bed. Everyone said that most patients would be mad. I just kept giggling and finally said "It's a good thing I don't have to go to the bathroom". Thay all started to laugh then. The therapist had to go give another treatment. He said he hoped they would not need a "beating".

Finally the maintenance man came and fixed the bed. Well, he thought he had fixed it. The whole experience was the joke of the floor the next day. The nurses knew I thought it was funny. So they were kidding me all day about it.

A few days later the same thing happened again. And it was with the same therapist at about the same time of morning. We could not believe it! This time the nurses had the maintenance man bring me a new bed. I was stuck up in the air longer this time, while he went to get the new bed. I still wasn't mad or anything. I just was not feeling so good this time. I could see that my therapist was really upset this time. Even more so than the last time. So I told him that I was going to skip my "beatings" during the nights from now on. He laughed and said maybe he should change jobs. But he is still there. I really got the jokes and funny remarks the next day. People said things like I would do anything for attention. We would laugh about it.

The thing about Saint Thomas is that it is a hospital that mostly has older, adult patients. So most of the other patients are really too sick to talk or joke around very much. Some of them would probably have gotten very upset over the broken bed incident. That's why the staff always tells me that they love having me as a patient, but they hate to see me sick. I always get the best of care. The nurses and everyone else always seem happy to do things for me. Some of my nurses have tried to get their patients swapped so they could have me again on their shift. I guess I have more friends than I think I do.

Each time I go into the hospital I stay about seven to ten days. When I get out I'm sore from laying in bed, and bruised from having so many different places stuck for an I.V. My veins just cannot hold an I.V. for more than a day and a half. The I.V. therapists were always having to stick me every day or so, and I really got tired of that. My veins are tiny and they roll so that makes it hard to get a good vein. But after a "tune-up" as I call each hospital stay I usually feel better for a few weeks.

As for Dr. Haynes, I could not have asked for a better doctor. He always makes sure that I get whatever I need. He really is a caring person. And he never hesitates to help me in any way that he can. I feel very lucky to have him as my doctor. I know that I never want to change doctors again, or hospitals either.

CHAPTER 11

Finally Some Help

I had gotten on medicaid because of so many medical expenses. I was needing more and more medicines. I was in the hospital so much more often. It got very depressing. My doctor said I would not get any better, and that I would need a steady means of insurance to cover the expenses.

Medicaid is not a steady means of insurance when a person is married and one of the couple is working. I was advised to seek legal help. If Jimmy made one dollar over the limit to make me eligible for medicaid, I would not get coverage for that month. It went this way each and every month. If I had been in the hospital during one of the times that I was not covered it was very bad news for us. What were we to do? How could I get help paying for my medicines? I had medicare, but that does not cover medicines. We were very worried.

I called around and got no help. Just one brick wall after another as usual. Many people that I spoke to were very rude and acted as if I were asking for the impossible. Even after

I explained my situation to them. One man I spoke to said that if I were to have a child, I would be sure to get all kinds of help. I told him that I wouldn't have a child if I could not take care of it myself. This was so unbelievable. I felt like I was losing my mind.

I'm not kidding when I say that getting any help with medical bills when you are not a child, a mother, or if you cannot afford a special policy is nearly impossible.

I decided to seek legal advice. The lawyers I spoke to said they heard these same stories time after time. The sick or elderly people who really needed help could not get it because of income or marital status. Many people choose to use welfare as a way of life; and this may be one reason why it is so difficult to give it to those who really need it. The system is so messed up.

When we asked what we needed to do in order to get help, all we got were some very sad looks. The lawyers I spoke to all said that they knew I could get help if I were to become single again. They did not tell me to get divorced to get help; but, the hint was there.

Jimmy and I decided to forget it and keep trying to get by like we had been. And I started to slack off on some of my medicines that we could not afford. I just got worse and then Jimmy and I would stay upset over the whole situation. We were so mad at the system for putting us through all this. It just was not fair at all. Our tempers began to flair up all the time. We were always at odds with each other over what to do. We talked to our families about what we should do.

Having to live with a serious illness like Cystic Fibrosis and worry about all of the problems that go with it was almost too much to bear. But to get a divorce in order to get help was making us very bitter against the system (and the world). When a couple loves each other so much, and they are trying so hard to get by, doing this seemed so tragic. We had no choice though. We filed for a divorce and got it. At least we didn't lie about it; we were not going to be able to live under the same roof the way we had been getting along.

After it was all done and settled we started getting along better. We had a ton of weight lifted off of our shoulders. We still never left each others side. We were still very much in love. We have been together ever since.

We have been together twelve years now. I would think that we have gone through more than our share of problems. We just want to be left alone, and enjoy what time we have left together. We have changed though. We have become so close to each other that we tend to close ourselves off from the rest of the world. Except for family members and a few very close friends. We are happier this way. And I don't think either of us will ever get over our bitterness at what we had to do in order to get help. We are not the only ones who have had to do this; we have since learned that it is becoming more and more common among the sick and elderly.

People take alot of things for granted. We are very grateful for alot of small things. Yet our lives are still a constant struggle. We still worry about every little thing.

Right after all of this stuff was taken care of we decided to move back home for the last time. We had been through so much, and we needed some quiet time with our loved ones, especially mine. I was absolutely worn out. The whole situation we had gone through really had me upset.

The cost of living in Nashville on one salary is not easy. The lease on our apartment was running out. That meant signing a new lease, with a higher monthly rent. There was no way we could afford to stay there. We had to find a more reasonable and quiet lifestyle in order to save our sanity. I told Jimmy that after this move back home, I would not ever move back to Nashville again.

CHAPTER 12

Going Home For Good

I went on ahead and moved in with my parents, just for the rest of the month. I needed some rest and relaxation before the move. The lease on our apartment was up at the end of the month. We had to find a place down home to move into, plus make sure it was ready in time. Jimmy stayed in Nashville at the apartment during those couple of weeks. I missed him so much I ached inside. I would cry myself to sleep at night. I was just so torn up inside about everything. I didn't know what to do.

Jimmy and I would talk on the phone every evening. Neither of us would want to be the first to hang up, so our calls were always sad at the end. I was with my family and that helped me some. And of course I had my poodle with me. Peaches is always a comfort to me.

I had to get Peaches groomed the same week that I moved home. I tried this one lady that groomed poodles, and she cut a place in his side about two inches long. She took him to get stitches and never bothered to let me know about it. I found out what happened when Daddy and I went to pick him up. I nearly fainted when her helper brought Peaches out to me. The lady that did the grooming never showed her face to us. It was probably a good thing, too. I was at the end of my rope. I went ahead and paid for the grooming, but I said I was not paying for the stitches or their removal. Thank God there is a wonderful place to get dogs groomed here now. Until a couple of years ago I had to go out of town to get it done. Now there is Kay and Dee's Grooming, Peaches loves the lady that owns this place. And it's only ten minutes from my home!

I will never understand how I kept it all together back then. I used to have long talks with my daddy. He was always able to help me figure things out and he always seemed to understand how I was feeling. He never had any doubt that Jimmy and I were meant for each other. If he ever doubted that we would be anything but together he never let me know about it. My mom did have doubts, and she mentioned them to me on more than one occasion. She would say things like "Jimmy won't have to stick around when the going gets tough", because we were not married anymore. Other people may have thought the same thing. They just never said it in front of me. I would always tell Mom that Jimmy and I love each other and no piece of paper (or lack of one) could change that.

Inside my heart was breaking each time she said that. I tried to be polite and just let her remarks go. But I did have my own doubts, I must admit. Afterall, I felt like I wasn't everything that Jimmy deserved. I will never forget a remark that a lady from the church we used to attend said to me once.

She said that it was a shame that I was such a burden on Jimmy. I'm sure she did not mean it the way it sounded, but I still remember the remark anyway.

One day I told Daddy that Mom was really upsetting me and I asked him to speak to her about it. The comments about my being able to count on Jimmy was stopped. By this time they had already slowed down though. We were all busy getting our new home ready to move into. Alot had to be done, it was left in such a mess. We got it all cleaned up and ready.

Jimmy was working days in Nashville and he would bring a truck loaded with our things home with him each night. He loaded all the stuff himself after working hard all day. I would help him with the light stuff, and Daddy helped him with the heavy things. We would work on the house until late in the night. Then we would rest until the next morning and start the whole process over again. It took about a week of this before we were all moved in. The truck was small and with Jimmy working and moving during each day (not counting the one hour drive each way), it took awhile to do.

Back at home me and my family were busy trying to get things in order. It was July and very hot out. When it was all finished we were all exhausted. We were finally settled in. Jimmy was really starting to look thinner and very tired. I was worried about him, but he said he was fine. He was worried about me and thought that I was looking tired. I was losing weight again. And I had been eating good home-cooked meals. I thought I would be just fine once we were settled. I ended up in Saint Thomas a few weeks later with my pneumonia again. The late summer heat and weeds that grow here always gets my problems stirred up. That's one draw back about the country life. I'm allergic to practically everything.

Naturally I was mad at myself for getting sick again. I had been so careful. Everyone was helping me so much and I was resting as much as I could. Why did this happen so soon? Nothing ever seems to go smoothly with us.

Jimmy still had work to go to, and now hospital visits with me. All with the same hour long drive to and from work each day. My hospital was in Nashville of course, so he called me on his breaks. Some nights I told him to just go on home and check on Peaches and rest. He didn't always listen to me, and he would show up for a quick visit after work. I would always cheer up when he walked into the room. He looked worn out, but he always had a smile and a big hug for me. He is a priceless person. I adore him. No one else came to visit me but him (like all the other times). I would cry when he had to leave. I always said that he had to give my poodle a hug and kiss from "Mommy" as soon as he got in the door. Alot of times he would call when he got home and put Peaches on the phone so I could talk to him myself. I could rest after that. No one ever questioned the love between Jimmy and myself after that.

It got to whenever I packed my suitcase to go into the hospital my poodle would jump into the suitcase and rake my clothes out. It was as if he was saying that he didn't want me to leave again. He is used to it by now, he is seven years old. He still gets mad when I start packing though. I am always with him, talking to him as if he is human; and he acts like he is most of the time. He knows about sixty or more words. We are very attached to each other (to say the least).

Peaches was a gift from Jimmy and his parents. I was really wanting a dog and they went together and bought him for me. He has been a blessing ever since the day we got him. And to say he is spoiled would be an understatement.

A couple of months after we had moved back home Jimmy got a job as an ambulance driver. We were so glad he had a job closer to home. He decided to take the course to become an Emergency Medical Technician, soon after that. He was always doing things for me and he felt like a healthcare provider already. The course to become certified was long and difficult. Jimmy passed it with flying colors. In the summer of 1988 he was certified as an E.M.T. We were very proud of him. He does this type of work very well. He has the patience and the ability to stay so calm during the worse situations.

Jimmy also felt like taking the E.M.T. course might help him learn more ways to help me during my bad times. A couple of times that I had to go to the hospital by ambulance Jimmy was working. That was really strange. Once when I was home and started to bleed alot, I could not get it to stop. Daddy called the ambulance and Jimmy and his partner came to carry me to Saint Thomas. Peaches was not going to let them out of our front door with me on the stretcher. Mom had to grab my dog and lock him in the bedroom. He was furious and growling at her and everyone around me. It's a wonder he did not bite her.

A few times when I was in the hospital and Jimmy had to make an ambulance run to Saint Thomas he would run up to my room. He could't stay but a minute while the patient he had taken to the hospital was being worked on by the doctor in the emergency room; but, just being surprised by him was great. I was always so proud to see him walk in my room in his E.M.T. uniform. He looks really professional in it. Cute too!

CHAPTER 13

Daily Needle Sticks

During the winter of 1988 I was sick (as usual) and in the hospital. This was getting to be so normal for me. Dr. Haynes said that antibiotics in pill form were not strong enough for me anymore. I would need them in the form of shots three times a day. Guess who got to do the job of giving me the shots? Jimmy of course.

My daddy had given shots to soldiers when he was in the army, but he said he could not stand to stick me. No one else wanted to either. So Jimmy learned how to give me my shots from a nurse before I left the hospital. He practiced on an orange and then the mattress. My shots needed to be given deep in the muscle that's why he practiced on a mattress.

After he had gotten the hang of it the nurse said he should do just fine. Then we were given a big bag of syringes, alcohol pads, and a prescription for medicine. Then I went home.

My first shot was due about an hour after we got home. Since Jimmy had not actually given a shot to anything other than an orange and a mattress, I was scared. While Jimmy was getting the syringe ready I was starting to get upset. When he started coming towards me for the big event, I started running the other way crying. I begged him to skip the first shot. After a couple minutes of this he put the stuff down and said so sweetly, "It's this way or back to the hospital". I gave in and braced myself for the pain. He was so gentle, I barely felt it. It was the first shot he had ever given and he did it perfectly. How could I have doubted his ability? Afterwards we hugged each other. We knew it was just the first of many shots to come, but I wasn't scared anymore.

This went on three times a day for a year. Then my muscles were like golf balls. We rotated spots for the shots from my arms, legs, and bottom. I preferred the arms. The only break I got from the shots was when I was in the hospital. After awhile, my veins got worn out. We had to find a way to get my antibiotics in me. I needed them everyday.

My doctor told me about a device called a Port-o-cath. It's a small, round disc with a rubber top on it. It had to be implanted in my chest; and in order to access it, a large needle had to be stuck in the rubber dome top. A big clear tegaderm would prevent the needle from moving around or coming out. Those needles were ugly to look at (they are curved so they won't come out easily). The needle had to be changed out every couple of days. And let me tell you, it hurt so bad to get that needle stuck in my chest. I did get some spray that helped numb the area, but it still hurt very much.

I had started having a home nurse come out to my home to do all the needle changes and give me my I.V. antibiotics. I would always take a pain pill about a half hour before she came to change the needle in the Port-o-cath. Just to prepare myself for it. When Cheri, my nurse, would pull the old needle out, she had to push down on my chest and quickly pull the needle out. Then she would clean the area and put a fresh needle in. We always prayed that the new needle would go in place and work the first time. If not, it all had to be done again.

It hurt, no doubt about it. But Cheri Markwell was the best nurse that ever changed that needle. We became good friends over the months. She'd talk to me to keep me occupied and before I knew it we were through.

I ended up learning how to hang I.V.'s and run them in myself. I needed my medicines four times daily around the clock. So it was a big inconvenience to always have her come out to my home that often. Before I learned to do them myself the nurses would take turns coming out to hang an I.V. They only took about a half hour to run the medicine in, so it seemed a waste of time for everyone involved to have them come out at all times of the day and night. I wanted to feel more in control of the situation. So I talked to Dr. Haynes about letting me do the I.V.'s myself. He was sure that I could do it, and I could always call my nurse if I had a problem.

Jimmy decided to take an I.V. Therapy course so that he could help me do things like figure the drips and stuff. He passed that course with flying colors just like we knew he would. He did everything he could to help me. And so did Cheri. Anytime I needed her I called her. She even said I could call her on her days off or during the night. She is a great person, as well as a good friend. As for being a nurse; they don't come any better than her.

CHAPTER 14

Hearing Aids And Diabetes

After a year of having the Port-o-cath in, it got worn out and badly infected. It actually grew to my skin and became one big sore. I kept it clean and dry at all times, but it still got so infected that it had to be removed. The doctors decided to give me a different type of device this time. I got a Hickman Catheter, which is a tube that is implanted in my chest and hangs out several inches. All I have to do with it is keep it clean and use an anti-clotting solution to keep it from clotting off. It's absolutely painless and alot easier to care for. I keep the tube that is extended out of my chest taped up and no one can really tell I have it.

I had to keep changing I.V. medicines all the time. The shots I had taken, and then some of the I.V. medicines I had used all had hearing loss as a side effect. We were aware of the side effect, but I didn't realize that I was losing my hearing. One day I was about three feet from the phone and it started to ring. Jimmy asked me to get it and I asked what he needed.

That's when we realized that I had not even heard the phone ringing at all. We knew I had been saying "Huh" alot, but it never occured to us that I was losing my hearing.

We told Dr. Haynes about it and he set up an appointment with a hearing doctor. As it turned out I had been reading lips most of the time that I was around people. If they weren't looking right at me I could not understand them. I had to get two hearing aids. The kind that go behind the ears. I call them my mufflers. But that is the kind that I need so that I can adjust the volume on them. My ears are sensitive to high pitched sounds. I have a loud ringing that is constant in both ears. That keeps me from hearing low sounds as well.

Peaches started telling me when the phone would ring by running to it and back to me, until I noticed him. I can hear some people on the phone better than others, but mostly I try not to use the phone because I just can't understand people on it. I have to ask them to keep repeating things. Peaches has trained himself to help me in many other ways. If something or someone is around the house he really goes wild. He keeps barking and carrying on until I go check it out. If he needs to go outside, he jumps up and down by the door until I let him out. People pay good money to get a dog trained as well as he is; I just got lucky and got a smart dog that learns things on his own. Another reason to love Peaches even more!

I have to be careful of the medicines that I use now. So many of them have hearing loss as a side effect. I can't use those unless we have no choice. I also have gotten so immune to many antibiotics that the choices are even fewer. The ones left I am allergic to or they just don't seem to help my type of infections. My life is always on a roller-coaster type of ride. There are always complications that have to be dealt with.

I got used to wearing my hearing aids after a few days. At first it was over whelming to me. It was like I could hear too many things all at once, it gave me a headache. Now I really benefit from them. People still have to be facing me in order for me to understand them. And I still have trouble on the phone, but I can hear better in general.

Then came my next hospital stay. This time I thought I would never get out of Saint Thomas. I was in there two weeks. I was supposed to go home one day, and on the day before that Dr. Haynes came in with more bad news. I had developed Diabetes. I was floored. I cried and cried after he left. The first thing I did after I was alone was grab a ding-dong snack (that I had in my drawer) and eat it as fast as I could. I was crying the whole time I was eating. A few minutes later a nurse came in to fill me in on what I was going to be going through. She checked my blood sugar level and it was high. I had to get my first insulin shot. I confessed to her about my eating the chocolate ding-dong after Dr. Haynes left earlier. When she saw how upset I was she said she probably would have done the same thing.

I kept crying until my eyes were red and swollen. I had to learn all about counting calories, diet, exercise, and watching out for sugar in hidden forms. I also had to learn how to stick my fingers and check my blood glucose levels. They taught me how to give myself insulin shots too. It was all happening so fast that I just about lost control. It was so overwhelming that I could not stop crying when I was alone in my room. They switched me to the diabetic floor in the hospital. I got a dreary, corner room. I was very depressed.

The diabetic doctor I started seeing was trying to figure out if I would need insulin shots daily, or pills. My having Cystic Fibrosis complicated matters alot, because I eat alot more than most people. And I eat more often. Being a diabetic meant that each morsel of food I ate was a factor in how my sugar levels would be. In other words; I needed to eat alot for the CF, but only 1,700 calories a day for the diabetes. The doctor finally decided that I am a type II diabetic (or non-insulin), I just had to be careful of my diet and exercise, plus check my blood sugar levels often.

I sat in my hospital room and learned all I could about having Diabetes. I watched videos about it and learned about nutrition. Learning about it helped me to cope with having it. My blood sugar levels act up mostly when I have a bad infection or have to be on high doses of steroids.

I learned to adjust my life around this obstacle. So many people say they don't see how I manage to keep my sanity with all that I have to live with. I always say that my sanity is questionable. Honestly though, I just try to keep a positive outlook and appreciate the little things in life. Being sick all of the time has made me aware of so many things that I might not otherwise notice. And I have Jimmy to help me through the rough spots.

They say you tend to marry a person most like the parent you love and admire most. I think Jimmy is a lot like my daddy. I can see so many ways that they are alike. Sometimes it seems like I still live under Daddy's roof. Because Jimmy has to baby me and spoil me most of the time. Jimmy seems to have picked up where Daddy left off. That's probably why I love him so much and fell in love so quickly.

Now all seemed to be pretty good for awhile. I was on my home I.V.'s everyday. I was feeling okay. When I got immune to one medicine, we would switch to another one. We thought things were looking up.

CHAPTER 15

My Heart Gets Broken

In the Spring of 1991, my daddy got really sick. He had always had trouble with his heart, blood pressure, and lung infections. This time it was worse. He went to the hospital for a check up in early April. The doctor found a spot on his lung and one on his neck. They found it to be cancer. Then he had to go through radiation treatments for several weeks. I watched this big, strong man become a weak and very sad person. We tried to hope for the best. We all thought he would be okay. But he had given up, his spirit had been broken when he was diagnosed with cancer. That was one word he never could say.

The radiation treatments were very hard on him. He lost so much weight and got to where he could barely move. He was so sick. One day after he had gone for one of his treatments he called me to say that he had good news for me. The doctor told him that he didn't need any more of the radiation treatments. They said the spots were cleared up. We were all so happy that we cried. We felt like we would have Daddy around for a long time.

He still had his lung infections that he needed to go into the hospital for I.V. antibiotics, but he had always needed them. We called them his "tune-ups", like we did my hospital stays.

A couple of months later (June 1991), Jimmy and I went to Florida for a few days. Daddy and Mom were supposed to go with us. They had never been to Florida. The ocean air is like a giant humidifier for my lungs; I always feel so much better after a trip to the ocean. We just knew that it would be good for Daddy. But the day we were supposed to leave he got sick. He called me and said he needed a tune-up at the hospital and we should go ahead and go without him and Mom. He said they would go next time. He was in a good mood and sounded fine. I didn't want to go, but he made me promise to go and have fun. So we left for our three day trip a little uneasy.

We enjoyed our trip and felt refreshed. My lungs were in need of the giant ocean humidifier. It worked like it always did for me, making me feel almost normal. And I did need a vacation. It had been a long two months and we were emotionally drained. But I could barely wait to get home and check on Daddy and of course to see my dogs (we had gotten an outside dog).

The minute we walked in the door I grabbed the phone to call the hospital. The nurse that answered the phone said Daddy was doing just fine. It was after hours for the patients to receive calls, so I told her to tell him I was home and that I loved him. She said she would tell him for me. A few minutes later the phone rang and it was Daddy. He sounded cheerful and said he hoped to go home the next day.

He had been home a few days when all of a sudden he started getting these knots all over his body. He went back to get them checked out. The way we understand it, the cancer had just sort of busted out all over his body. It wasn't supposed to be that way at all. The treatments he had were supposed to help him not make the tumors go crazy. We don't exactly know what caused it, but he got sick again really fast.

One day he was walking with a walker and the next day he was in bed unable to get up. Then Mom got a wheelchair for him. It was like a bad movie that I wanted to stop watching. A bad dream that I wanted to wake up from. Only this was real. I was falling apart at the seams watching my beloved Daddy slowly die in front of my eyes. I could not stand it. I refused to believe what was happening. I was going to make him fight to live. He could not give up, I needed him. I loved him too much to go on without him. I told him to fight, to draw strength from me. I was at his bedside every second that I could be. I was afraid that he would give up if I left his side. He seemed so frail and quiet.

His birthday was coming up on June the 17th, and the doctors had sent him home to be in more comfortable surroundings. It was a very hard time for all of us. We were used to celebrating Daddy's birthday, Father's Day, and my birthday (June 21st), all on the same day with a big cookout. This year we all sat around the living room watching Daddy slowly eat ice chips (that was all he could hold down). The silence in that room was as thick as a brick wall. Everyone was just crying and watching Daddy.

The next day I decided to make a cake and fry up some chicken. Daddy loved my fried chicken. I took him over some cake and a couple chicken breasts. He ate them like he was starved. Which, I guess he was, since he couldn't hold down food for long. I felt so good seeing him eat. I felt like he was going to get better afterall.

A few days later he was back in the hospital again. He was getting worse. His attitude was better about things. He would be cheerful and smiling one minute, and in a deep sleep the next. It went on like this all day long, each day.

On my birthday Daddy called me first thing in the morning. He always wanted to be first to sing Happy Birthday to me. I cried so hard as I listened to him sing. He changed the ending of the song to "Happy Birthday, my sweet baby". I nearly collasped as I listened to him. I knew I would never hear those words from him again.

We all stayed together as much as we could. The family as well as some friends of my parents. It actually seemed like there were too many people just sitting around. Most of the time Daddy was resting and was not even aware of what was going on around him. I would have liked to have had more quiet, family only time. But my opinion was not well received. Mom, my sister, and I took turns staying with Daddy all of the time. None of us wanted to leave his side.

Daddy was sleeping all of the time so he would not feel any pain (he was on a morphine I.V.). One afternoon I was sitting beside him telling him what we could do if he would hurry up and get better. Then I said I loved him more than life itself. I was just sitting there when all of a sudden he squeezed my hand three times. I was holding his hand and watching him. I knew he heard me when I told him that I loved him, because he did squeeze my hand. That was a signal he and I had been doing since I was a little girl. Whenever we had been in a place like church; where we had to be quiet, I would say "I love you" by squeezing his hand three times, and he would squeeze back three times.

Mom insisted it was his reflexes, I knew better though. I asked the doctor if Daddy could hear us talking to him and he said yes. Mom and I seemed to drift farther apart after that. I could not understand why Mom would be so upset at me for trying to talk Daddy into fighting to live. She and her friends from her church were telling Daddy to "Go towards the light", so I was actually going against her in some ways.

Mom and her friends were always in the room carrying on conversations about things, when I walked in they would say I had to be quiet. I was being shut out of the last few days of my father's life by complete strangers it seemed. If I could not talk to him in a soft soothing voice, how could they all sit there talking loud enough to hear in the hall? It made me upset but I kept quiet.

When I left the night of June 25th, I asked Mom and Sheila (even the nurses) to call if Daddy woke up or if anything happened. It was getting late, and I had not eaten all day long. They were afraid I would get sick too. So I said I would go home and eat. I kissed Daddy bye on his cheek and told him that I loved him and would be back later.

I left the hospital at 8:20 p.m. and at 8:32 p.m. I was heating up a microwave dish of spagetti. It exploded in the microwave and at the same time I felt like something was awfully wrong. I went to the window and looked out at the night sky. There was this big, bright star out that I really hadn't noticed when I came home. I knew that if anything had happened at the hospital someone would call. They had all promised me that they would call. I still could not shake the feeling I had. I forgot my dinner and went to watch some TV. I was too scared to call the hospital myself and Jimmy was at work.

An hour later, Jimmy came walking softly into my room. I never heard him come home. I didn't have my hearing aids in. I was just sitting there crying when he walked in. I could not understand why he was home so early from work. I remember asking him if he had quit work since he was home early. He sat down beside me on the bed and grabbed me. I was screaming so loud that it better not be about my daddy. I was hysterical and so much in shock. I knew what had happened. Jimmy said that Daddy was not hurting anymore. I demanded that we go do something, try CPR or something. Jimmy said it would do no good.

We went to the hospital to see Daddy and let it sink in that he was gone. The nurse met us at the door and gave me a pill to take. I went in to see Daddy and then back out to be with my family. Only my mom seemed to want her friends around her more than me. So I went in the chapel to sit with a friend of mine that worked at the hospital. Jimmy was helping our friend that owns the funeral home here take care of Daddy. When I asked my friend what time my daddy had died, she said 8:32 p.m., the exact time my dinner had exploded in the microwave.

I felt as if our souls had touched when Daddy passed away. He always promised that he would be my guardian angel when he died. To this day I have this warm, calm feeling that comes over me when I'm really upset or have alot of problems going on. It seems like Daddy is saying that everything will be okay. And it usually works out that way a day or so after I get that feeling.

I used to hear Mom say that after I left home, on some nights Daddy would just wake up out of a sound sleep and sit up. When she asked him what was wrong he would tell her that his baby was sick. Meaning me of course. The next morning he would call me early to see how I was, usually his feelings were right and I had been sick during the night.

We had his funeral and my heart was broken. I could not understand why I was always having to hurt so bad in so many ways. Daddy was my best friend, and he never hurt anyone. He was the most wonderful man I have ever known. I was on the verge of a nervous breakdown. My doctor had put me on valium to help through this awful time. I passed out right after the funeral, when we went back to the house and I noticed Daddy's empty chair. I realized then that I was alone except for Jimmy.

Jimmy had so much to do already, how was he going to care for a heartbroken Daddy's girl too? My life was never going to be the same again. I gave up on living, I didn't care about anything anymore. I wanted the hurt to stop and I wanted to die.

Jimmy had his hands full. He tried to carry on as usual. But he was hurting inside in his own way. He and my daddy were very close. He had to take care of me, and put his grief on hold. I just lay around and stared at the TV. I did this for several months. My family was of no help to me at all. Sheila had my niece, Jenny, to try to get through this hard time. Jenny was also very close to my daddy. As for Mom, she took comfort in being with her friends from her church. She spent alot of time with Sheila and Jenny as well. But when it came to me, Mom just didn't have the time to come around. It felt like I had lost both parents. Mom rarely came around to see if I was okay. She even mailed my birthday card the following year instead of dropping it off as she passed by my home. She has been dating a man from her church for several months. Some people say that it may be because I was so close to Daddy that Mom feels strange coming around me while she's involved with someone. I cannot understand why she still acts so cold towards me, though. I have not said anything against her dating or her lifestyle. That's her business. I just want my mom to act like a mom should act. I need her love and support, even if I am thirty-one now. I finally dealt with losing Daddy but I can't seem to deal with losing Mom, too. She is very close to my sister and niece, I am sure that she always will be.

I have an older sister, Jane, that lives in Illinois with her family. An older brother, Kris, that I haven't seen in years. And my brother, Terry, lives out of state too. The rest of my relatives live in Illinois, Indiana, and Florida. So my whole family is scattered out pretty far. Mom doesn't have much to do with any of them either. I just never understood how a person could just write off her own family members the way my mom has seemed to do. I wish I could understand. When I ask about it, Mom says she is too busy to do things with me. Yet, she finds time to be with Sheila and Jenny. I'm not crying sour grapes here, I just do not understand what happened between us. We used to be such a close family. Since we lost Daddy, everyone has gone in different directions.

Sheila and I have remained close. My niece, Jenny, is a very special little girl to me. We will always be pals. She always tells people that her Aunt Debbie loves her more than anything. She has always been like the little girl that I could never have myself. Our relationship will always be special to me.

So, other than Jimmy, Sheila, and Jenny I guess I'm pretty short on nearby family for support. Jimmy's family has always been special to me. I know that if I need them they will always be there.

CHAPTER 16

Life Goes On

During the months that have went by I continued to do my own I.V.'s at home. I still didn't want to depend on my home nurse to come and run the medicines in for me. I was having to mix the medications myself; not an easy task to do either. Jimmy and I would sit for an hour or so at a time mixing enough medicine bags to last a couple of days. This saved me time, so I could just hang the bag and run the medicine in when it was due.

We got supplies by the boxes full. Our spare closet was for supplies, not extra clothes. I had syringes, tubing, I.V. bags, alcohol pads, tape, gauze pads, gloves etc... You name it and we had it. I had to keep up with every bit of this stuff, making sure I did not run out of something. It was aggrivating as it could be, but I had to have the I.V.'s in order to get by. Some life, huh?

I could have just sat back and let my home nurse do the work for me, but I would still have to keep up with the supplies.

And I could have gone into the hospital each month for the antibiotics. I was now only getting my I.V.'s one week out of the month, unless I got sick or something. My lungs were not really any better. We were just running out of antibiotics to use, so we had to use them sparingly. Hopefully I wouldn't get immune to them that way. Even though I did not feel like doing all this myself, I did it. I still wanted to feel somewhat self-sufficient.

In June of 1992, Dr. Haynes decided to try a different antibiotic on me. One not available in I.V. form. I was so glad. Maybe it would do some good. I wanted to stop having to do all the I.V. stuff at home. The medicines I was on had stopped helping my infections along time ago. I was so tired all of the time. I did not have the energy to keep doing the things I had been doing. I could not even take a shower without getting completely exhausted. I have so many coughing attacks now that I can barely do anything. I have to rest between showering and doing my hair. There is no way I could do my own I.V.'s like I used to anymore.

Just breathing is about all I can do myself anymore. I feel almost like an invalid. We are not sure if the antibiotic I'm on now is helping me or not. I have so many different types of pneumonia germs that need to be cleared up. Just one pill doesn't seem to do much good. The antibiotics that could clear up my problems are the ones that cause more hearing loss. So we cannot use them unless we absolutely have to.

I cannot seem to go more than four hours without my aerosol now. If I happen to be a few minutes late with it, I can tell. I'll be all wheezy and tight in my chest. Then I'll start to cough and choke. It's awful to be this way. I was this way even when I was on home I.V.'s so we knew that they were not working then. The newer medicine I'm on still helps some, but we are waiting for something new to come out that will help me. There's a new drug called Dnase that I have heard alot about on TV, my doctor said that he has high hopes that it will help me when it becomes available to the public. It has not been approved for general use yet. I can hardly wait to try it. I need help fast. I don't have any choices left for help to keep my lungs clear of infections. I feel more desperate as time goes by.

This past June, we went to Florida for a few days. My doctor thought that it might help clear out my lungs like it used to do. I was so sick and worn out that I had a hard time during the drive down there. I was bleeding some and having bad chest spasms. I was using pain pills and codeine every few hours. After we finally got there, I was feeling some better. But not like I was used to the ocean air helping me feel. This time I still felt congested and ached in my chest. All the other times we had been close to the ocean I felt like I could breathe so far deep into my lungs. It was such a cleansing type of feeling. This time I felt just like I had been feeling at home: sick and worn out.

We still had fun and enjoyed ourselves. We just did things slower and less of them. We rode out on a cruise boat and saw two dolphins chasing the boat. That thrilled me to no end. I adore dolphins. We went to see a dolphin show at this one place and they even let us pet the dolphins. I could have died right then and been happy. I never even dreamed that I would get to do those things. When I first saw the dolphins that were going to perform at the aquarium I lost control of myself and started to cry. They were just so beautiful and graceful. We took eight rolls of pictures on our trip. I would say six of them were used on those dolphins.

I have often said that when I die I want to be cremated and have Jimmy toss my ashes into the ocean so I can be close to the dolphins that I love so much, and the ocean.

After we got home from vacation we were out in the yard one afternoon. Out of no where came this little dog. It leaped right up in my arms and started kissing me. It was like it had known me all along. I had never saw the dog before that day. At first I thought she might be trying to bite me or something. We asked the man next door if it was his. She had evidently been hanging around his store for several days. She wouldn't let anyone near her.

She sure seemed to like me and Jimmy. He pulled ticks off of her and cleaned her up (she had fleas). I got some food ready for her. The poor baby was starving and thirsty. She had came to the right place for love. She acted so scared and lost. We tried every way we could think of to find out where she belonged. No one knew of a missing dog. She is a house dog, but with Peaches being inside I was not going to let her in unless I knew she was healthy. We kept food and water out for her for a couple of days, thinking she would go home. But she was always by the door with that sweet face of hers, wanting in. We decided to let her in and later take her for a check-up to make sure she was in good health. By now we were in love with her. She is so smart and loving.

We call her Candice Paige (or Candy, for short). And she is now a proud member of our home. I just love her so much. We have a good time playing, and just watching her.

The vet said Candy is one good little dog. She is a mixed Terrier and about two years old. We got her shots and headed home that day. Wondering if we could handle two dogs in the house. The first night we let her in, she decided she wanted to sleep in the bed with us. We let her, because Peaches sleeps on the bed too. How could we make one get down and the other not? Candy is totally housebroken (thank goodness)! She rarely ever has to go outside. We really were blessed when we found her. Well, she actually adopted us I suppose you could say. Like Peaches, if she needs to go out she will tell us.

I put real newborn baby undershirts on both of our "babies". We have a big guard dog in the backyard, we call him Casey. So even though we don't have any real kids, we do have our special kind of "babies". I even put all of their names on Christmas cards and letters etc... This past Christmas we got cards from my friends and family, they put "the Pitts family" or they added each dogs name on the envelope.

Now when I go into Saint Thomas Hospital I really do have alot to tell all of my friends. Plus, more pictures of my children. Some people might think that I am crazy. But I have an addictive or obsessive type of relationship with Jimmy, as well as my dogs. It keeps me focused on living.

CHAPTER 17

A New Year Means New Hope

It is now January 1993. I was hoping to get this catheter taken out of my chest, but I doubt if that will happen. I have been really sick for the past three weeks. I got sick before Christmas. I wasn't able to get out of bed because I was so sick with a fever, coughing, throwing up, and I even started to bleed again. I haven't bled from my lungs like this in quite awhile. It brought back bad memories. I'm on higher doses of steroids and a different antibiotic, but they are not helping at all. I know I'll end up in Saint Thomas, so I have my bags packed. My coughing spells are so bad that Jimmy has to blow in my face to give me air after I finish coughing. I feel terrible, I just want some relief.

I did end up in the hospital for eight days. I had to take two different types of antibiotics that will effect my hearing. We had no other choice but to use them. I have so much infection in my lungs from the pneumonia germs I carry that it will take awhile to clear up. I am too sick to worry about the hearing loss from the I.V.'s. My bronchitis is in full action too.

One morning in the hospital I was having a bad coughing spell, I called for my nurse to bring me a codeine. While she was gone, a cleaning lady came in to clean my room. I was coughing and gasping for air. The lady asked if I was going home that day, I said no. She emptied the trash and started to mop the floor, I started to cough harder. My face got really red and she looked startled. She asked me what I had that was making me cough. I said Cystic Fibrosis, but it was my pneumonia and bronchitis that was really acting up. She literally ran out of the room. She never finished cleaning or even said goodbye. She just left. I felt a little bit like an outcast.

My nurse came in a second or two later. I told her that I had scared the cleaning lady. She smiled and said she knew already. The cleaning lady had stopped my nurse and asked her why I wasn't in isolation because of my having so many things wrong with me. She was really scared of the word pneumonia. My nurse told her that we were on the pulmonary floor and more than half of the patients had pneumonia; and it was not contagious anyway. Then my nurse apologized for the behavior of the cleaning lady. I said it was okay, afterall I am used to people being scared of me. I told her that I even scare myself sometimes, and we laughed. People can't help it if they get scared of someone coughing so hard that they turn red in the face. I do sound bad when I cough, and when I'm really sick it is even worse. You can't blame them if someone gets scared for that.

I did get to see all of my friends (respiratory and nurses). We got to catch up on all the latest stuff. I made some new friends too. One new respiratory therapist I met used to work with CF children when she was in training. I figured that she could answer some questions I had about CF that I never asked anyone about. She said if I had the guts to ask them, she would answer them.

I wanted to know how most of the CF patients that she had worked with before that had died; lived their final days. She said that they were kept as comfortable as possible with oxygen for breathing and morphine for pain. Then, she said, they just drifted off to sleep and that was it. It was very peaceful and quiet. The patient usually was so sick that they required hospitalization every couple of weeks, as well as being on home I.V.'s. So that means they were alot worse than I am, I suppose. At least my question was answered.

I have always worried that I would be gasping for air, bleeding alot, or in alot of pain when I die. I still might be in one of those ways. But I try not to think about it. My medicines are narrowed down to so few now that I can't help but be afraid of the inevidable. I just pray that some new antibiotic comes out that will help me. And that the new drugs waiting for the FDA's approval will be available soon.

If I don't make it long enough to try it; I hope that other people with Cystic Fibrosis will be helped by it. We have to suffer so much and hurt so bad. Dealing with this disease is hard enough, but having to go through all the red tape to get help for older patients is just as hard. Waiting on the red tape to go through and new medicines to be approved is too much for some of us to handle on our own.

During my eight days in the hospital this time I was busy putting the final touches on my book. I was so upset and depressed about being in the hospital that I could not rest good. When I did get the chance to sleep, I was awakened coughing my guts out. Many mornings I was sitting up at two o'clock wide awake, looking out the window at the night sky, waiting for the sun to rise. Many nights I would cry myself to sleep, exhausted from coughing so hard.

Our best friends surprised me one Saturday night with a visit. Debbie and Roger Atkinson with Amy and Corey (their kids) popped in to bring me a plant. Debbie brought it in because kids are not allowed on the patient floors at the hospital. Roger stayed by the elevators with Amy and Corey. I had been so depressed that day, Jimmy and I were watching television when Debbie came in my room. It made me feel so good to know that our friends care enough to drive over an hour from home to visit me in the hospital. I walked down the hall (pushing my I.V. pole) to see the rest of my visitors. I think I surprised them by meeting them. I just had to go see them, I missed my friends so much. I wanted to hop on the elevator and head out of that place whith them when they left. I knew I had to stay though.

These are really the only friends we go out with. On the weekends we try to go out to eat either Friday or Saturday night with them. Thank goodness neither of them smoke. We go looking around a store or two and then back home. They have the sweetest kids you could ever meet. I love them. I can be myself around Debbie and Roger, they know all about my problems. They understand what I have to go through and they really care. I consider them the best of friends. I also know that "if" anything should happen to me, that they will be there to help Jimmy through it all. Otherwise, Jimmy would suffer in silence.

I was glad to get home from the hospital, and we all went out to eat a few days later. Just like old times. I still was not feeling so good, so we took it easy. I was sad, Dr. Haynes told me that I will probably have to go into the hospital every couple of months for the same I.V. antibiotics that I used this time. I have so many germs in my lungs that we are going to need strong medicines to keep them from growing. I sure don't want to get this sick again, any time soon. But, the thought of more hearing loss doesn't thrill me. We know that will happen with the medicines I need. Dr. Haynes said that all we can do is wait for some new medicine to become available. Until then it looks like our choices are limited. I'll do whatever I have to in order to live.

I was in a store today getting some typing paper, and I started coughing so hard all of a sudden. People started looking at me like I was a freak or something. I dropped the paper and ran to the bathroom, which happened to be closeby. I wasn't sure if it was the employees restroom or not. I didn't really care at that point. I just got in there and coughed until I cleared out and got control of myself. Then I went back out as if nothing had happened. Jimmy was waiting for me, and we just left after that. I get so tired of this happening.

I have had people offer me cough drops, or make some comment about my having a terrible cold or allergy. I just say whatever I think of at the moment and get away from them.

CHAPTER 18

My Thoughts

When someone has a life-threatening illness, they may do some risky things sometimes. Maybe just to prove that they can or cannot do them. Maybe just so they can do them before they think their time on earth may run out. I have been guilty of all of these things. Some I have regretted doing. Some things I have done may have hurt me in some ways. But taking chances and making mistakes has made me what I am today. Sure my quality of life is not very good, I just can't seem to do very much of anything on my own anymore. I just try to think of the positive things that I have done in my life. I concentrate on holding onto what dreams I have for my future (however long that may be). Mostly, I just wait for a cure to be found for this horrible disease of Cystic Fibrosis.

I dearly love Jimmy and my dogs. My friends and family mean alot to me too. Jimmy is my life line though. Without his love and support I would not be alive today. He puts up with all of my mood swings and crying spells. Mostly he puts up with my always feeling so bad. I've been this way for so long that he doesn't really see the real me anymore. The "me" that wants to get out there and do things like everyone else does. I guess he will never be able to see that side of me again.

I have talked alot about Jimmy in this book. I have told you about the way he helps me around the house, and how he takes care of me when I'm really sick. He does alot more than his share sometimes. Yet, he never asks for anything in return. He is such a good, kind-hearted person. I owe him so much for all that he does for me. All I can give him is my unconditional love.

Each time I get sick, Jimmy gets scared. He doesn't like to show it. I have known him so long that I know when he is worried about something. Jimmy always thinks that I will bounce back after a bad spell. I used to think he was mad at me when I got sick because he was so quiet and withdrawn. Now I know that he gets this way out of fear. He is afraid that one day he will lose me. I don't know how to comfort him when he gets scared, we both know what will probably happen one day. That's why we try to be together as much as possible. I just wish so much that we could forget all about medicines, doctors, infections and everything else and just go away for that special honeymoon that we never did get. One day maybe we will. One day maybe all of our problems will be solved.

Our lives are ruled by things that we can't control. We accept that and take one day at a time. We never forget how blessed we are with the love and friendship that we have. When it comes down to it; that's what life is all about.

While writing this book my life is going through so many changes. I'm really tired and so worn out. I feel like I am alot older than I am. My body outside looks normal still, but inside it feels like it is twice my age. No one can seem to help me right now.

My friends say that I am too good of a person to have all of the bad things wrong with me that I do. I ask myself what I ever did to deserve all of this, sometimes. And then I think about all the love I have around me, as well as the love I had while growing up. So many people aren't lucky enough to have that these days. I guess things are not as bad as they seem then.

This book may sound awful, or hard to believe, maybe even sickening in some parts. But every word of it is true. I live it and feel it each and every day. I cannot just read this book and say "Oh, that poor girl has a rough way of life". I have that "way of life". I don't want pity from people. I just want their friendship and understanding. Most of my friends are in the medical profession of some type, so they understand what I have to go through. That means alot to me. They think I handle things really well. But, I still live in my own little world.

There are not many books out about Cystic Fibrosis. I only know of two of them. I always try to read up on how other people with CF live and manage from day to day. What they do different than I do etc... So many people aren't even aware of what Cystic Fibrosis is. And it's been around for years. Of course not too many patients live to be very old, maybe that's one reason why CF is still not well heard of by most people. You mention that you have it and get a puzzled look. Maybe this book can help in some small way to inform a few more people about what Cystic Fibrosis is and how it effects people.

The next steps are new medicines becoming available for us, some form of health and life insurance, and most of all a cure for us. I pray for the day that a cure can be found.

I just cannot stress enough how much a positive outlook is for a CF patient. We all have a big battle to fight just to breathe each day. It never gets easier for us. With the right attitude and a good outlook; plus lots of love from family and friends, maybe we can live longer happier lives. It has worked for me so far. Great medical care is absolutely necessary. Find a doctor that will work with you or your child. Make sure that you and your doctor have a good relationship. And whatever you do, never give up the fight.

Life is far too precious and too short, so appreciate the small things. If you were handed lemons, like I was, you can make your own lemonade.

I hope anyone reading this has a full and rich life. If you have Cystic Fibrosis, or just know of someone who does, may God bless you and keep you healthy.

CHAPTER 19

Some Good News

It has been almost a year since I wrote this book. So much has happened during this time. I thought I would update things some.

I have been taking the experimental CF drug called DNase since May. It really does seem to be helping me keep my lungs clearer. I don't have any large amounts of energy or anything like that; but it does help me. I am also taking my antibiotics in large doses with my aerosol pump, instead of in IV's now. Along with all of my regular aerosols I usually end up taking about eight treatments everyday.

A couple of weeks ago I had to have my gallbladder removed. It was really scary for me since they had to put me to sleep to do it. It took two and a half hours for the surgery. I am just now starting to feel like my old self.

Last week Jimmy was offered a job that he has been trying to get for over eight years. This means that he will be gone all week long for training. He can come home for the weekend, then back for more training. All of this will go on for about three months or so; then he will be assigned a specific county to work in and we will probably have to move. The field of law enforcement has always been Jimmy's dream job. Now his dream can (and is) coming true. The thought of moving and exciting changes being made is a little scarey for me, but I'll be fine.

The CF drug that I mentioned, DNase, has been approved by the FDA. I heard it on the news last week. Now many more people with CF can try it out! I heard the good news after I came in from shopping the other day. I was so tired, I had not been able to get out much before the Christmas holidays, so I tried doing too much at once. I hope that it didn't wear me down. There are alot of colds going around and today I am congested more so than usual. Of course I'm not getting my extra "beatings" since Jimmy's in school. I'll be fine though. I take extra precautions to make sure of that.

I got a beautiful bracelet from Jimmy for Christmas. It has fifteen gold dolphins that surround my wrist. I just love it! He got me a crystal dolphin figurine, too. I look at them and feel such love in my heart for Jimmy and my special friends of the sea. I got other things for Christmas as well, and I love all of them. I also got a watch that has a dolphin swimming around the dial of the watch, from my sister-in-law and her family. That really is cute. There is just something so free and innocent about a dolphin, it must be the reason that I have always been so drawn to them.

Speaking of dolphins, my mom and her fiance' were married in Florida before Christmas. Bob is a great guy. They are down around the Florida Keys, where there are places that let people swim with the dolphins. When Mom called to tell me the news, I told her to kiss a dolphin for me if she swam with one. Can you imagine the thrill of that? I would probably pass out or something.

So, all in all the new year shows great promise for us. I am feeling better since I got my gallbladder out, Jimmy has gotten his dream job, my mom and I are close again. All we can do is keep on doing the best that we can, and hope for the best for everyone.

I made my new year resolutions the other day. I'm going to try to keep my positive attitude for another year. I really would like to stop being so superstitious. And if I can, I wish I could stop worrying so much about the little things in life. I can't forget to keep fighting this CF either. That's a big resolution that I make each year. The last thing is to show the people that I love, just how special they are to me as often as I can!

3-31-94
10:30 P.M.

On the morning of 3/30, early, I was saying a prayer like I always do out loud. I asked Daddy to please help me feel better and help keep me out of the hospital. I was really feeling bad and had a fever. I was congested and nauseated too. But I first asked him to please keep looking after Jimmy (and me) and help Jimmy through this last week of school because I know it will be a busy, hard week. I asked him to help Jimmy pass his tests too. I said please and told him I love him etc... As usual. Then I said I wish I could get a sign of some kind. To let me know he heard me.

I could remember him always saying to me to always do my very best and everything will work out fine. I thought that was my sign. I told Daddy that I loved him, again and ended my prayer as usual ---

About 15 or 20 minutes later my big heart balloon that was facing the window (had been all week long and only moved if I turned the fan on or something) slowly started to turn around so the words I love you, was facing me. I was trying to go back to sleep but I was awake and saw the balloon moving around slowly so I watched it. After a couple minutes it went back to the way it was before –facing the window. <u>That</u> was my sign. I know it.

At lunch time I was taking aerosol and went to the sink to rinse the nebulizer out – I noticed my balloon was facing the kitchen at an angle, where the words I love you was showing again! I said out loud I love you too Daddy. Later on it stayed turned the other way the rest of the day and I was in bed all day too. I would have seen it. Today it's been turned around facing the windows all day just like it has been all week except for the 2 times it turned around. It's sort of scarey, but then again I know my prayers are being heard. Now I guess things will be ok. At least I hope so! I'm going to try to stop worrying so much. And just believe it'll be ok.

4-28-94

As I sit at my kitchen breakfast bar I can see out my windows looking at our big backyard. I love this place, it's so pretty and quiet yet it's not far from town so we never have very far to drive when we need something from the store. Let me start at the beginning.

Jimmy, my husband of fourteen years, was sent to this town after graduating from the police academy. We knew nothing about this county and thought we'd never find a place to build our home. Finally one day Jimmy found six acres at the end of a new subdivision. He drove me over to see it one Sunday since it was his day off. I was so upset. "No way am I moving here", I told him. I was thinking that he'd have to move here without me and I would stay at our other home alone. He could come home to me and our dogs on his off days.

The six acres was completely covered with weeds, trees, rocks and I could only guess what else. It looked like the woods and I'm definitely not that country. Afterall, I'm originally from the big city. I cried all the way home that day. I begged Jimmy to do something else. He promised he'd try. But he said that the land in our new town is very expensive because of a new car plant that was built a few years ago not far from here. Jimmy could see big things in those six acres. I could only see weeds.

Just after we got back to our other house I called up my Mom and my sister. I cried on their shoulder and told them I just couldn't see myself moving an hour and a half away. Let alone to "the woods" as I called it. But I reassured them that Jimmy was still looking for something more our style. Especially since I had refused to move if he didn't.

A couple of days went by and as Jimmy began his job of learning the roads and riding the county with his training officer he scouted the area for land to buy. The houses we looked at were all very overpriced, so that was out of the question. Each day Jimmy would come home elated from work – he loved being a state trooper. He had always dreamed of being one. But when I asked about a home or some land for one he'd shake his head and say "sorry babe".

"What are we going to do" I asked? We had less than two months to get some final decisions made and plans started. We knew what we wanted and all we needed was a place to start.

I'll never forget the day Jimmy came in with a sly grin on his face and a piece of paper in his pocket. "What did you do now?" I had to know. But I was also afraid of his answer. He smiled and said "I bought us some land

and they are going to start working on it tomorrow." I couldn't believe it. Where, how, and why without asking my opinion I thought. But he seemed so happy. I smiled and said "great, where?" That's when his smile faded. I sat down at the table and said "no, please say you didn't by those woods?" "But listen," he said softly, "it's really going to be beautiful." "Have I ever lied to you?" Well, he had never really lied. Stretch the truth maybe but not lied. So I tried to act happy. He filled me in on all the details.

He had trucks hauling in dirt after he had them clear off all the land. Then came the septic tank, light poles, contractors were coming and going for days on end. It was hectic to say the least. I was at our old home while Jimmy drove back and forth each day to work. When he worked nights he went in early to make sure things were being done on time. He really took charge of things. I was so proud.

On his days off my step father helped clear off alot of trees and move some things over that we could do without until we moved. They made a place in back of the property to keep everything safe and out of the weather.

Meanwhile we sold our old home and the lady was going to move in the day we were actually moving out. It was a holiday weekend so it would be easier on her and us.

So Jimmy tried to speed things up. He got his Dad and brother to help. They worked so hard. They built a fence in the back yard for our dogs and more. And once it was all ready I could not believe my eyes. Our six acres is not only cleared but we've been living here over a year and I love it. Sure I miss my family and our long phone conversations. But we have a gorgeous place here.

Jimmy and I hand sowed our entire yard with grass seed after we moved in. Then we put straw over it to keep it moist and to keep it from blowing away. The first few months we had mud for a yard and our 2 house dogs tracked mud in whenever we let them out. We kept a bucket of water by the back door to wash their little feet off but they still got muddy. Our big outside dog still gets upset because he misses our deck that we had at the old place. He used to like to lay by the door and watch us. Here he's out in his pen with just his doghouse. He likes to run and play in the yard though.

We finally have birds here too. For the longest time we didn't see any at all. We put out bird feeders, a bird house, even a bird bath. Now I get to fill up the feeders all the time because we have tons of birds. Squirrels, rabbits, and a deer I call Annie started coming up in the yard the other day. Now I feed her lettuce and vegetables. I guess you could say we have quite a place here. We finally have a big beautiful home. There's always something to be done. We had to buy a big riding lawnmower, a chainsaw, even a fancy weed cutter that really does a good job. I am amazed at how Jimmy can work for hours on end just keeping our land cleared and looking beautiful. I do what I can, but our house keeps me busy too.

It just goes to show you that when the man you truly love promises you that he won't let you down. There's a good chance that he means it. If he loves you like my husband loves me.

In the meantime we want to build a deck and maybe later put in a pool. I can look back at the pictures Jimmy took from time to time as our place was being turned into our beautiful home. Those woods sure did end up looking pretty good. It goes to show you that some people can see beauty in everything. I will too, from now on. Like when Annie comes up in the yard for her salt block or vegetables we put out for her. Or when our baby bunnies hop all over the yard and play around the blue bird family that just started living in their bird house. I can sit for hours and watch our yard and feel full of pride at what we've accomplished and how lucky we are to have our place and each other.

As for Jimmy's job; he really is happy, finally. It took a long time before he got his dream job and he's doing wonderful.

We miss our family and friends that we left behind. We see them often but you know how it is when you get to feeling blue and need cheering up. I haven't made many friends here. Everyone we know works all the time so it's pretty much the two of us. And our dogs of course. We'll be fine and we have really gotten to know each other even more if that's possible.

1-20-97 – 2-1-97
CAME IN ST. THOMAS

1. Psneudomenas pneumonia (from culture)

2. CAT SCAN shows "sinuses" infection "BAD" and deformed bones in left nostril. May require surgery to correct; but first we'll do irrigation because of lung condition at present.

3. MRSA – staff infection grown out of sputum sample. Requires a very special anti-biotic; since it is very resistant to all others. Except like 2 I'll be on the strongest of them. Now also – being isolated from people.

4. IV's not lasting long with all these strong meds/laryngitis side effect too.

5. 25th. Started the bleeding from lungs again. Very irritated this time.

6. Started nasal irrigation 1/26/97 – will need to do this 3 times daily twice with another anti-biotic solution. More stuff to mix and keep up with. Not real comfortable to do. Gave me a bad headache.

7. Swapped IV sites again. 25th less than 24 hrs.

8. More bleed peak and traugh – not easy to get.

9. 1-26. My IV's are no good. Gotta get a pick line or central line. Put in ASAP.

10. No voice above a whisper. Maybe from aatrovent aerosole. By the way, nasal irrigation going ok. Works great. A water pick will be good.

11. 1/26 – 12:30. Gotta get IVs redone now. May quit with blood returns and it is puffing my veins up as you look at it! I need more bags up till AM so it'll not ease thru this tiny bad vein. Then we go for the biggy vein tomorrow.

12. Please God and Daddy help me thru this.

13. 28th. Things are crazy! Was gonna get a pic. too much for my arms to take. Veins are *all* hard and dry. Trying to get'em thru till *Sat.* When I hope to go home. As far as the rest – lungs are ok. MRSA is not clear yet. Sinus wash makes me sick but it's ok. The food is awful. Got wrong orders. *BAD* roast beef, and even mold on my bread last night. Finally got "part" of the order after 8 last night.

14. 29th. My latest iv is ready to be swapped! It is so sore. Not in for a day yet! Couple more days to go. Don't know how long this will last! I'm so nauseated from this med! *Ranky vank!!* Ribs sore from hitting it yesterday on tray.

15. Really tough day! IV's acted up. Already had to swap out one from yesterday. Had a bad reaction to "vank" today. Had to get phenergan 2 times. Dry heaves, pale, very bad feeling. Blurry vision. Retha had a feeling I needed

her just as I was! She restarted IV and got an extra one to carry me thru. She's off tomorrow. Amazing how she felt that I needed her. She's real nice. I think alot of my problems now are from too much juices. Sugar levels are bound to be high. Need to go home bad. Dr. Haynes says Sat. man that's far off. Especially bruised and sore at 1 am. My arms look awful. Coughing up really icky stuff. Seems like vank and Fortaz make me groggy and nauseated.

16. This stay seems really hard, can't and won't let myself get so bad next time if possible. Only it's the staff infection that is making me so sick. The "Ranky vank" is so awful. But the food is really bad. So I drink alot of pop, and juice and eat alot of yogurt to help my dried up esophygus. I can barely talk above a whisper. Although a few good things have come out of this. My relationship with Mom and Dad has flourished. I could not have made it without them! Period. They have done so much for me. Too much I feel sometimes. They come here every day. Mom pampers me and mothers me. Dad just does whatever needs doing with a smile on his face. Lord have mercy – how could I ever have faced this without them? Because Jimmy had to work. It's been a true experience and a test of love and strength. I think we passed the test. They've been great. Got beautiful Dolphin figurine from Mom and Dad! You've never seen something so beautiful. I love them.

17. IV's still in both arms. We're going on a cruise. I'm gonna focus on that. Jimmy and Dad wanna go. Jimmy deserves a treat now. I guess it'll be in June. But me

and mom are gonna buy a major economy size box of Dramamine. As for the kids, I can't worry about that. A cruise is a once in a lifetime thing. And I'll go – I have to start living a little more. Doing more for those that I love and that love me. Sitting home praying not to get sick (and being a loner) makes life boring. So – I'll pray and do things carefully. Sounds like a plan. Hey – mom and dad treat me like a queen you know? Well, they left yesterday and Jimmy came to see me. I look awful, but I'll do better. My idea is to get this facial swelling down. Just checked back-up IV—it's good for today! Anyway – after I ate my favorite Arby's Cheddar beef Jimmy brought me last night here came supper. A good one for a change. So I ate it too! Then we snacked around on fruit etc... I got meds (Fortac and Imep) and sleepy so I know it was high sugar I could taste it. But Jimmy fixed me a yogurt and him one. We ate more. He smiled more, talked to Lynn too. Then later I dozed off so Jimmy went and got 4 juices, 4 cups of ice, a coke and filled my (thank the Lord for cooler!) with fresh ice. He caught one yogurt with it's date up 18 days ago in there. It got in on my supper tray. Anyway it's a new day. My heads hurting bad. I wanna take a nap but I did my nose and can't lay back yet. I'm sleepy. Miss my family wanna go home and curl up with my fiddly dee. I'm hungry.

18. 30th. Still Dr. Haynes took me off "vank". We found out that it hurts my ears and makes me real sick. Put me on more pills. Lowered steroids to 20 mg. 8 hrs. So, I can still go home Sat. Got Hayes (the nurse student) to copy side effects of Vank, Impepon, Fortaz. We saw the side

effects of Vank: and Fortaz and it makes me too sick. The Fortaz makes my vision double and blurried. Something is making me very sleepy and I can't function or think straight. Vertigo it's called.

19. Yes! My nurse from the first night has been in again. Stock up on food. Mary.

20. 31st Friday. OK A.M. but had reactions to Fortaz. Had to get phenergan again. Feel some better but still sore. Wayne brought me a real genuine Starter NFL Dolphin sweatshirt!!!! Cannot believe it! Just for nothing. He said his son needed one bigger and instead of swapping it he thought of me. Still in shock! Makes me thankful to God for all my friends and family that helped me thru this. It's magical. The love and compassion that people have for others. It may not be a perfect world or a healthy world that I live in but: my Mom and Dad along with Jimmy and my friends here at St. T. I made it thru a long tune-up. Now all I gotta do is rest more. 15 days more of isolation at home. My arms look like road maps purple ugly road maps. Mom has massaged me 'till her fingers cramp I'll bet. It helped s<u>oo</u>o much. And today I had to have another IV changed and Dad couldn't get to my hand because they pulled one as they stuck the other hand! It hurt too! Now it's supper and Jimmy's off for a cookout steak! My supper stank but it's ok. My chest is spazzing out BAD. Well, going down off steroids fast and from IV solution to pill prednisone. It started hurting about 6. Some lady's choking now real bad. She needs to get her butt in her room and close her door. This is the

pulmonary floor and that's how I got staff infection for goodness sake. I'll be so glad to be home. I'm gonna miss Mom and Dad everyday though. What will I do then. It makes me cry now, but I will be ok. Maybe they'll come see us alot. I can't go there. Least not for 15 days! Still makes my heart smile when I think of all they've done for me. How can I ever show them how much I love them? Thank God for good parents!

21. SAT. Going home. I'm so glad. So sore and tired. My legs are weak I have a hard time walking. Can't wait to hold my kids. Crawl into my bed. See my house and appreciate my things.

22. Last night did the craziest thing. Got up to go to bathroom, headed towards front room with imaginary IV pull and it got stuck. Woke Jimmy up yelling for the pole to move I had to go to bathroom. He said I didn't have the IV anymore and go to the bathroom to the left – I was asleep. Then I was sleepwalking again and was trying to unplug the IV machine at the head of the bed. Woke Jimmy up pulling on the headboard he had to wake me up again and steer me towards the bathroom. Then I asked for apple juice and yogurt. I ate and drank it. Didn't remember anything. Crazy huh.

23. Can't sleep at night for more than an hour or so. I get up and snack. I am sooooo skinny my legs don't even touch at all except at the knees. My bones stick out. I look so bad. Because of no food in the hospital. I'm nearly starved. Can't think, see straight, remember anything much. I'm

so weak. So tired. Need lots of help. Mom and Dad are coming to see me Tues. Miss 'em – can't wait.

24. Had a pretty good day. Enjoyed our visit. I got showered, did my hair and felt pretty good. I vacuumed with my red Devil vaccume Jimmy got me for early Valentines Day. I love it.

25. Rough day. Started to bleed <u>bad</u>. Lots of it. Sore and achey. Can hardly move. I'm scared I'll end up back at the hospital. Cannot stand the thought I'll carry <u>bags</u> of food and pop if I do that's for sure. Sometimes I wonder what's gonna happen to me. Sometimes I just don't think about it. But I can hardly get around I'm just so weak. Never felt this way. Now I need meds. for the bleeding to stop so I'm having a hard time seeing and writing and everything else. I'm tired for now. I did do a load of laundry before I got sick today. Can't do much of anything. Probably won't be able to read this either.

26. It's been 6 days since I got home and I'm still so weak. My legs don't feel right. They won't move like I want them to. If I bend down I have to pull myself up with my arms still. I have a good appetite though. I eat nearly hourly round the clock. Me and Jimmy are doing fine. We had a talk the other day about "stuff". We admitted we were scared. I'm still bleeding though alot. I finish Bectrim anti-biotics tomorrow! They are so hard to take. They hurt my stomach. And I'm sore still. I wanna find out more about this MRSA infection. I can't find out about it. I cough more and more. Is this the beginning of something

else. Know what I mean. I have so much to do. So much to say. I'm scared. Last night the show ER was about a kid with CF and the ER had a staff infection going around! Go figure! I was coughing up blood watching that I was shaking so bad I couldn't wait for Jimmy to get home. Then I couldn't sleep. Why? That's what I wanna know. I squated down to get a magazine and couldn't get back up. I sat in the floor 10 minutes I know my arms couldn't pull me up the edge of the bed was too high.

27. Having a tough time on low steroids! Miss 'em. Need 'em. I'm addicted to them I know. I can't move without aching and actually hurting all over. Still look terrible. Legs and arms are so – skinny. I slept 'till like 4 or so today, then got up for yogurt and codeine. Bleeding a little so I stayed up. Then back to bed at 6:15. Bad thing to do! I over slept till 8:30 or so and medicines were late. So it threw my steroids and aerosole off. Been goofy all day because of it. I'm tired of being sick! I'm tired of aching! Won't it ever end? I wanna be ok again like last summer. It was so nice. I was tan and healthy feeling. And happy. Now I don't feel good and I'm so give out. Who am I writing to anyway. Jimmy, Mom, Dad, who? Who ever you are – if I'm not around hug my dogs and tell them their mama loved them ok. If you can. And if I'm not able to hang on – I hope they are doing ok without me. I spoiled them so much. I shouldn't be thinking what I have been through but I'm afraid the ole swan song may play if you know what I mean. Mom and Jimmy say I'm just worn out and been thru so much. And I have hope that's what it is. But if not I'll be able to rest and breathe until then I'll write when I can and keep notes on this awful tired feeling. MRSA. It

STINKS! Whatever it is. CF too! It's not fair and it hurts and I'm mad at it 'cause I'm tired of everything. Hey, Kathy (the groomer for peaches) says that sinus surgery helped her brother.

Feb. 10

28. This morning I slept till 5 o'clock. Woke up thirsty and my mouth hurting. Coughing too. Jimmy had to work days. I could've went back to bed. I tried, but I coughed too bad got up did my nose thing with water pik. What a rush. It's tough, but if it helps ok. I prayed alot too 'cause I hurt in my chest so bad. I got doped up. Ate and did some laundry. I'm slow but whatever. Had to make appt. to see Dr. Haynes and Dr. Courey too on 24th hope that's ok with Jimmy. I'm tired of doctors! I'm about fed up all together if I don't start feeling better I'm gonna bust! Writing it down helps sure but lets get real here. I took some albuteral today. Maybe a little won't hurt. I hope it doesn't. It helped open me up some. I needed that. I want to feel better so I may have that sinus surgery. Everyone says it is awful (for 2 or 3 days it's real bad) and after a couple weeks of bed rest a person feels better. Everyone is able to breathe after that. I don't know. I guess I'll find out on the 24th. If I can breathe better it may be ok. "If" Mom would be able to take care of me afterwards. Only if she could 'cause I know Jimmy would be busy and I'd need babied. He's always busy and he's not much of babying. Hopefully by the 24th Mom and Dad will be close to coming home if I do need surgery. So it'll work out ok. We'll see.

29. Things are the same here. I'm still not feeling good! Still
can't get up if I squat down for anything. My body aches
and I can't breathe! I'm mad and I can't take much more.
Jimmy is really starting to get irritated. He's been snapping
at me for 5 days now. Every little thing I do or don't do
bugs him. He tells me I have an attitude problem. I don't
think so. Even if I did though – I'm entitled I think. I
cut down on steroids to 20 and man I can barely move
in the mornings. By 2 or 3 I'm ok. Then by bedtime
I'm tired. But this business with stress is making matters
worse. If I hear "if you are so unhappy you know what you
can do?" one more time I may just leave. I'm so fed up. I
cannot ask for one lousy thing, or say anything without
Jimmy jumping down my throat yelling I'm never happy
and I always want something. That's a lie I don't bug him
for anything. If I want something I get it myself. If he
gets me something I thank him. Too much he says yeah,
right. I feel so lonely and like a burden to him anyway. All
he ever does is gripe about what he wants to do or what
I can't do etc... And he is *always* saying stuff about other
girls. It doesn't make me jealous. It plain hurts. If I say
anything then I'm hard to get along with. Nevermind
my feelings. Inside me there's a carefree young, healthy
girl. Just waiting to be set free. I want so bad to be that
way I try. But it's just not possible. Now Jimmy looks at
me and makes a face like he's disgusted – he'll say he can't
hug me or get close because I'm to skinny or too sick.
But he can still carry on about other girls and doesn't
care one bit how it effects me emotionally. It's verbal
abuse. He's always done that. Sunday night he started an
argument and I just went to bed and said I wasn't going

to fight. He said good, or else I'd have to call you a few names. He's always done that too. I don't need this. I love him; but I have to think of me now. He's ok. I'm not. I talked to Mom tonight. I really miss her. They are talking about getting central heat/air when they get back from Florida. I told her I may go stay with them. Extended stay. Jimmy doesn't want me here. I know that. I couldn't tell Mom that though. Everyone says me and Jimmy are the perfect couple. If they only knew. He really despises me and I've never did anything to him but love him. He's always thought I am no good or beneath him. Now that he's a trooper its gotten worse. He won't admit it. But it's true. The things he says to me are bad, lies, and hurtful. Things he's made up in his mind and he believes them. Why I'll never know. But I have stood by him all these years. He's gone thru alot of crap and I still stayed. I've gone thru alot of stuff too. But I couldn't help mine. His stuff was mostly his choices. Until he got his trooper job I always said it'd be the end of "us". It may well be. We've been going in circles for a couple of years now. No matter what I say or do – he wants the opposite. He'll pick a fight on the most perfect day out of the blue for no reason. Then he'll start in on me about me being so miserable. Why don't I just leave. I have no where to go. But now I might. He'd better be careful about what he wishes for. The other night after 8:30 he came in to "see if I was ok." Yeah right! He brought Karen Russell in to show off the house. Now the bathroom light was on and he could see that from the driveway. Yet, here they came walking in. I could've been on the toilet. In fact I had been about 10 minutes before that! Imagine if I had of still been. He never said anything just walked in with this goofy blank look on his face saying "you ok". I was so surprised that he'd bring someone in and not tell me. I started telling him stuff when Karen walked in and said Hi there. I didn't even get mad. Not a little. If I had been on the toilet I would have been so embarrassed and mad too. But since I wasn't it was ok. Still it was very inconsiderate and rude I think on their part. He's always doing things that are thoughtless. I say something about it and we argue like today. I had an awful time up till lunchtime. Then I asked him to go get some BBQ wings from Bi-Lo. He told me off in a heartbeat. Said cook some myself or make do with something else. It was sprinkling outside so I should have known he'd never go. But I didn't feel like cooking at the time, my wings weren't thawed and I was hungry. That's when I said he didn't ask me yesterday if I even needed anything from town when he took peaches to the groomers and went to pick him up. He yelled – if you want something speak up or forget it I'm not gonna ask you all the time. I said I just did ask for something (the BBQ wings) and was told I always want something blah , yeah, blah ... He didn't know what to say. He wanted some stuff for his truck – expensive stuff that's mostly for looks. But the Lt. and Trooper Logan got a bed cover for their trucks so he had to order one too. The truck is pretty the way it is. No less – he's been on this kick for over a week. And he ordered the thing yesterday. Now who sounds like they are never happy? He still wants rails for it.

30. Well, I've moved into the guest room. I was up mad, stressed out and coughing at 1 o'clock still so I said forget

it I'm going to make the guest room mine. I changed sheets, reversed the comforter and took my essentials in there. This bed is great. I put an afgan under the fitted sheet (why I don't know) and it made it feel like a warm set of flannel sheets or electric blanket was on the bed. I didn't sleep good though. I coughed alot. And my left arm is like so numb. I keep shaking it but it feels like it's asleep. Who knows. I'm deciding on if I should bring the kids in here too. I don't think I will. (Leave them for Him to enjoy). I knew what Jimmy's major problem is. I am 100% positive. He wants to date other girls. He's hanging out with guys and other single people who poke around on girlfriends and fiances and whatever the crowd is doing Jimmy wants to do too. Only I'm in the way. That's why he always tells me to leave if I say one single word against anything. No matter how insignificant it may be over it was because I ran out of room to hang his uniforms up to dry. I made a statement like I wish I had a bigger laundry room. And he blew up. If you don't like it here....well you get the idea. Now that I'm sick people ask about me, or say tell me Hi etc...It seems to bug him too. He doesn't give me the messages unless I hear him talking and he'll say I'll tell her. Then when he doesn't I'll ask him what it was. Mom can say what she wants. I love her and Dad so much. Ok – maybe Jimmy's scared. But move on with life. Enjoy the days we have if we can. Why does he have to continuously pick fights? Why does he always have to carry on and on about every single girl that he sees on TV and in real life? And above all why does he talk about them to me as if I'm a locker room buddy? I'd rather not know or do I care about big boobs or whether someone could quote "Rock Your World in a Major Way". Think it if he wants but shut up already. Believe me I fix up, do my hair get dressed in jeans and a nice shirt. Does he notice. No. He won't hold my hand if we go somewhere either. He put on a wonderful show of caring when we lost Grandma. Everyone was impressed. Even me! Then on the way home not 5 minutes out – he started an argument with me. I had said it was nice of John to drive all the way there after working all night and without sleep to be with Lee. Next thing I know I'm being cussed out because no one else I know would have done it for me ---- meaning the same old story. He doesn't know what he's talking about. He just went a couple days without being nasty so he had to get his digs in while he could! He had no conscience or manners! I was bleeding from the lungs before we got out of KY! Thanks to him. I'll be better off if I leave I know it. Lord knows he'll be happier. I've already sort of padded the blow to Donna. In a long letter I sent her the other day. If I can't get out of this misery one way I'll try another. I wish my arm would wake up. My chest hurts too.

I'm almost done with isolation! For all the good it does me. I still don't feel like going anywhere. My vision is so bad I'm scared to drive. But when I leave I'm taking my Blazer. He tricked me into trading my car for it. The payments are double my car's. But it'll be ok for awhile. I'm not giving it to him or my liscense plate Ted gave me. I've told him already that it's mine and I want it on my Blazer. He laughs and says it looks good on his truck. Screw him. I'm getting it, it's mine.

In the meantime I'm here trying to make do 'till Mom and Dad get home and get central heat put in. At least I can hope can't I. And plus Mom can give me postral drainage without griping about it too. But she's a mom. That's what Mom's are for right?

31. Well, I'm doing better today 2/14. I'm getting used to being on low steroids I think. I cough so much more and I wheeze so loud. Sort of like before I went in the hospital. I feel like my pneumonia is still there. I can tell. I didn't get alot of sleep last night. No wonder I'm so messed up. Jimmy says it's my meds. I don't think so. Not now anyway. I'm on such a low dose anyway. Unless it's my pain meds. Could be that. But still I'm going nuts here. I can't take much more of this. Jimmy got me a dozen roses and a beautiful card for Valentine's Day. After all we've been thru all week. I just can't figure it out. It could be his work and stress. He usually picks fights with me when someone complains about a ticket. He got a call from the post while he was in town but they didn't say anything. When I told him he said he wasn't worried about it. They could leave him a message on his desk or call him at work if they need him. Which leads me to think that someone must be acting up and he's bothered by it. He doesn't ever tell me straight out about things. I have to find out the long, hard way. Usually like this. Whatever it is just tell me. I don't like going thru the grapevine and being chewed out for something I had nothing to do with. At all. He got me all kinds of goodies at the store too plus the In Style Feb. issue I wanted. So I guess he feels guilty about something. I wish I knew what. This has become more

of a diary/journal huh? Maybe it'll help me get thru this. Oh yea – some great CF foundation. They never called back. How rude of them. Maybe they'll send me some info. about MSRA. I doubt it. Did I write that Mom called last night? They're in W. Palm Beach Florida! I told her things were difficult here and not any better. And I asked her to get me some turtles candy! She said ok. And I told her I'm not feeling much better and I may go live with them. She said ok. I wish so hard things could get better. Health wise and relationship wise too. This stress is giving me a migraine!

32. Finally the last day of isolation. Really it's tomorrow I think. But I probably won't go anywhere anyway. I look as rough as I feel. I do need a haircut though. I got up early today coughing. I took aersoles and inhalers, and meds. then went back to sleep for awhile. I got up later ok and made pancakes. I only ate a couple small ones so my sugar doesn't get high. Me and Jimmy are speaking at least. So things are ok. He came home early last night mad, cause Logan took another Friday off. The others just won't work Friday nights! They leave it for Jimmy to work alone. That's unfair. Actually they aren't supposed to even take Friday off. But Jimmy hung around, we had popcorn and soda and watched TV. Until I got sleepy and started nodding off. Then I came to bed. He had to stay up and wait to clock out. Anyway – I'm doing ok on 20 mgs of steroids. Gotta go to 10 on Mon. I think. Don't wanna try that . It's awful to think about. So I won't. It's a pretty, sunny morning. That should cheer up alot of people!

33. Had a good day. Got out and went shopping! Got new bed linens and comforter for my room. New houseshoes for me and gym shoes for Jimmy. I saw the most beautiful pocketbook. I wish I'd never seen it though. It's 50 whole dollars! Way too much. I'm not worth that much of a price tag. It's a stone mountain purse that's why. I was slow walking. I hurt in my hips and legs real bad. My joints hurt. Steps are too much for me to use. But I made it all thru the stores and mall. I am tired. We ate at Arby's and had a nice time. Jimmy was gonna get a new TV for the bedroom with closed captioning. Service Mdse. was out of Magnavox TV's all together. That's what we were gonna get. It's a good sale. They have some at another store if he wants to go get one. See I really save money if I stay home. But then I'm also bored and depressed. Everyone needs to shop sometime. It's been one month since I've been in Wal-Mart or any store. Until today. I have alot of making up to do. Maybe if I shop and exercise more!? Then my legs will get more limber. I hope. We were gonna see a movie too – only the one theater doesn't let troopers in free and the other one we always go to was so packed we couldn't get in. So we said forget the movie for today.

34. I almost went to my regular bed with Jimmy tonight. Glad I didn't – we were up 'till nearly 12:30. It's 3 now and I'm up coughing! I turned over in bed and started to cough. I'd hoped I was over all that. What am I going to do with out my stuff? I'm keeping this so Jimmy or Mom can add on to my book with clips from it or me even. My book. What a joke huh? It's like the only way I can get it out there is to copy it and pass it around. Then someone

reads it and says – you should publish this. Yea right. Easier said than done. Publishers say different.

How come we dream goofy things? And in our dreams we're normal? You know what me being up means don't ya? I'll oversleep in the morning. Or else maybe I'll be like the other day. More cleared out. Anyway I hope I am not cranky. You should see these house shoes I got. They are like suade boots really. All suade uppers, rubber soles and flannel lined over the ankles. I think they're like $20. I paid 4 for them. They had more. Mom will want a pair I'm sure. We got 5 tubes of toothpaste w/free tooth brushes. Because they were 1.49 each. And we have like 25 or 30 tooth brushes in the cabinet. We saw Crystal who cuts my hair in the shop at the mall. She was busy as usual. But she permed her hair. It was so cute before. Now it's loose curls covering her head and flopped across her face. I think it looks too dressy/modelish for her. What can I do about that purse? Jimmy offered to half it with me. I want it so bad. I can't get it off my mind. He's right – I do always want "more". But maybe I'm right too. Wanting makes us normal. That's about as normal as we well, me myself can get. About the cruise business. We are supposed to find out about it and book one for 4 people the 2nd week of June. Jimmy, me, Mom, and Dad. They might as well have switched condo dates from Feb. to June. Cruises mean money down, bookings, and all that way in advance. I don't like putting money on something so far in advance. You can't get it back or maybe just some of it. Whatever. The way I feel inside with my lungs and my bones I'm not sure if I'll even be around in 4 months. I hope I will and all. But you never know. I really would like to go on a 3 day one. We'd have to drive (or fly) to some place in Florida and go from there. And leave my Blazer for 3 days! Now that is another worry. Jimmy's Dad and Donna wants us to go somewhere in Mississippi on a gambling boat or something. I'm not sure, they took Todd and Kim already. I don't like gambling unless I win. Money is hard to come by. I suffer so much for mine. If I was so into tossing it around I'd have gotten my purse without a second thought. Call me thrifty. Call me cheap. Jimmy can spend money on things without hesitating. Me, I think it over and over ... 'Till I decide one way or another. When he spent $100 bucks maybe more with shipping and handling on that truck thing the other day I told him then and there that I was gonna get myself a stone mt. purse no matter what. I guess I lied. Right now I'm nauseated. I took a dramamine. I need a phenergan. I'll have to get one. I was so afraid of germs Sat. at the store and mall. I'm still coughing alot and I really have to walk so slow. I wish I at least could be more normal. The way it is I look sick. I'm under 100 lbs. I know it. I asked Jimmy to massage my legs and he said they were all bones. No meat to massage. But he tried anyway. What's going on here? I'm eating like a lumberjack most of the time and I still look like a boney skeleton. Here's what I look like naked ok. My knees touching – standing naked – my inner thighs like about 4 inches even to touch – my shoulders and ribs stick out, my arms and legs are about the same size, my legs are some bigger but not much and my stomach only sticks out a little. Not attractive *AT ALL*. Scary is what it is. Plain ole scary. Jimmy says he thinks I can eat all the fattening stuff I want and not gain any weight. He said he believes I'll always be too skinny no matter what. He was just saying it. Not to be mean or anything. Actually he's been real nice since Valentines Day. He snapped at me about not resting and I snapped back. Then he got nice and stayed that way. I wish we both could – be nice to each other most of the time. I really do love him. He just has a hard time accepting that or believing it. I'm not sure why. Maybe 'cause he grew up on his own without any praise or a loving set of parents. That's gotta be it. Material things always makes him happy. Hugs or holding hands or an I love you would do the trick for me. I'm not hard to please. I have a slight feeling he may offer to take me to get my purse today. It'd be like him. I wish I could get my eyes to focus! – More later as usual. Maybe walking through the mall will ease the soreness outta my bones! Too!

35. Today was great. We went to Hickory Hollow and I got a really cute purse. All leather for 20 bucks. Then Jimmy said he was gonna get the stone mt. one for me but since I found one I liked he didn't need too. Well, they had one made just like the Stone mt. one only in a taupe color. I want a black all occasion one. So I am looking at Wal-Mart stores for it, or else who knows I may still want the other one at Dillards. We fixed my bed up together. I ironed the bedskirt and we made it up all nice and pretty. I got a comforter and new sheets that actually fit. Dolphin color and yellow. Man I wanted to sleep in my other bed with Jimmy though. I fell asleep on the couch as usual. I'm coughing my head off and hurting bad. So – I'm in "my" room. We debated about it. Then I really coughed

alot so we said forget it. If this keeps up I don't know what will happen with us. There's a closeness, a bond that's not right anymore. Like we're strangers or brother and sister. When I hugged him goodnight it was different. Sort of sad. Maybe because all my babies are all in the other room and I'm alone. Like in the hospital. I'm so fed up. He got us a new TV with close captioning for our room only. I can't use it since I'm in here. That makes me mad. I cough so much on 20 mgs. of prednisone that I'm not going down to 10. No way. Everyone says don't. I had a spell in Target today coughing like a fool. Had to hide in the linen section and then go to the bathroom fast. Just like before when I went in St. Thomas both times lately. I'm gonna surprise Dr. Haynes with a spit cup since I have 6 of 'em (sterile ones). He'll ask for one I bet. Anyway – I was fixing strawberries tonight and Jimmy was feeding Casey, the phone rang 3 times I heard – I grabbed a napkin and dried my hands to get it. Caller ID said it was Lynn. Only he hung up and didn't say anything or so I thought. About an hour later Jimmy said his Dad had left a message so it rang 4 times and the machine was turned down so I never heard him say anything. Didn't see it blinking either. But he left a message of some sort. I don't know what. Jimmy called him back but never got an answer. Who knows. I'm so tired. I'm wheezing so bad and yes I do need postral drainage. I'm not gonna ask for it. Things are tough enough and it's late. Guess I'll try to sleep.

36. Feb. 17, 3:30 A.M. up coughing and spitting again. My mouth is sore so I ate some yogurt. Now I'm taking aerosole. This albuteral may be too strong but I sure

think it helps. I'm so scared of losing Jimmy. He's really buckling under the pressure here. We talked about lung transplants – he agreed that he probably couldn't/wouldn't stick around and watch me go thru it. I already knew that. And now he's doing about the same thing with all this. I just don't think it's fair at all. Who said life is fair anyway. But this getting up and down at night is wearing me out. I fall asleep every evening after supper. Every night! He has to watch TV alone during the day too. Cause I fall asleep mid-morning and after lunch. Usually one or the other. I'm just give out I stay cold most of the time even though he has the heat turned up to 70. It stays on alot too. God please help me get better. Let's do something to make me feel better. Please. I just want to be ok again. As for a cruise It'd be fun. But I'm not sure about going anywhere like this. I'm just not sure.

37. Woke up at 7 to an awful noise. Candice Paige was crying. Not a puppy dog cry but a bawling kind of cry. I thought I was hearing things at first, then I realized it was her. Making the noise she makes when we leave her alone at the kennel to go on vacation. It's a wail more than a cry. She realized her and peaches was alone I suppose. In their bed, after Jimmy went to work. The poor little thing was scared. I ran as best as I could to let her out. I wish she could sleep with me in my room. Maybe Jimmy should let them out when he goes to work and they can get in bed with me. That way I can get some more sleep. Otherwise they are probably gonna wake me up like that again. We'll have to wait and see I guess.

38. I trimmed my own bangs. They were getting so long and heavy. The rest of my hair needs trimmed too. Don't know when I'll get to go to the mall again. It wore me out Sat. and it was crowded. Too long of a wait. I'm so tired now. I could take a nap, but Jimmy said we're going to town when he gets home. I've gotta look at Wal-Mart for that other black purse. The one that looks just like the one I want at the mall. Man I wish they'd have one over here. I really want one. It was so soft and buttery leather. The one I saw was taupe but surely they have 'em in black and other colors I hope. If not and they have one (any color) I'll get it. There's something going on with my hips, and legs. My right one especially – still can't get up if I stoop down or if I try to walk up steps and have to use one leg and hold on. Like a baby does. It hurts constantly in the middle of my hip bone. Like I've been kicked or punched in the leg area. Its not from my phenergan shots or else both hips would be the same. In fact my left one is still real bruised and its not sore. But if Jimmy goes to hug me and pats me on the bottom – if he does it to the right hip it really hurts bad. I feel like my legs have lead weights on them when I try to walk like from the car to a store. And sitting down then getting up forget it. It is uncomfortable. I wonder what it is. Sitting in the bathtub is something else too let alone getting in and out of the tub. I was fine 'till the 2nd week of my hospital stay. Then I started getting stiff legged. We thought it was because of me being in bed alot. But I'm not so sure now. I wonder if Dr. Haynes will be able to tell me what it is.

39. Went to town with Jimmy. Stopped at Big B for some meat. The jerk in there got smart with me about one of

my prescriptions. Hopefully he's just a substitute guy. And plus, it took way over ½ hour for 4 things to be filled. I was so mad. We were gonna go to the teller machine and Wal-Mart. But we skipped Wal-Mart. Then everyone chose tonight to call and see how I am so we basically missed Melrose place.

40. Woke up with a temp. 99.5. I'm so cold though. The heats on high. But I've got on a flannel gown, sweatpants, housecoat and house shoes plus I'm under the covers. I'm bleeding again. Not mouthfuls though, not yet anyway. We want to go see a movie when Jimmy gets home. I'm coughing so bad right now I'd not step into a theater to see anything. Why does it have to be this way. Why? I'm *SO* miserable. God never gives us more than we can handle. Right? Well, for how long is what I need to know. I cannot take much more. Really. I've begged to get better. I've tried everything, followed doctors orders to the "T". Nothing is helping me. I'm so tired. My head is splitting and I can't get cleared out to breathe. I'm on 20 mgs. of steroids. No way can I go lower I need air. Now. Either help me out here Lord or else give me some rest. I can't do it on my own. It's just not fair. I've never hurt anyone. And I live in a private jail. And my family suffers too. Especially Jimmy. It's not fair to him. He's trying to buy a bass boat by the way. Oh he's mentioned it a time or two. Motorcyles too. But last night he was in negotiations about trying one out before he buys it. I couldn't believe it. His Dad has it, it belonged to Derrick in Florida. But even if it's a great deal with a good powerful motor – why do we need it? We rarely go anywhere. It'd be fun sure.

But it's alot of money! Even if he's letting Jimmy have it for just what he paid for it. I have to pitch in every month for part of the Blazer payment. If Jimmy's so anxious to spend some cash make my part of the payment every now and then. That'd be real nice. Then I could shop more. I need to quit that anyway. What's the use. I can't go places. Oh yea. I cut my own hair yesterday. The top and bangs only. It had to be done. Now all that needs doing is side and the back and blend it all in! If I ever get to the mall again. With me wanting that purse still – Jimmy will probably avoid the whole mall area for months! But when we turn in our bonus points we get a $5 off certificate. That wouldn't be till next month though. And they'll probably not have the pocketbook then. Who knows. I got a great one the other day and I love it! So if I don't get the black one (which I need) I'll make it anyway. Did I write about me weighing myself at Sv. mdse. on Sunday? 100 lbs. with clothes and purse and jacket whew. Oh hey, you know what else? I have no appetite anymore. I want stuff. Then when I get it I'm not hungry anymore. Like last night. Fried chicken, bake potatoes, bake beans. I ate ½ a potato and nibbled on the chicken. Not sure if Jimmy noticed or not. I'm just not hungry. If I could breathe I might be hungrier. That's neither here nor there. All I do is add stuff to this crazy journal. Who's it for anyway? My heads busting. I made myself eat some toast and jelly for the sake of my morning pills. But I cooked 2 pieces and ate most of it. I'm so sleepy. Gotta snap out of it and go to town. Maybe at least let the kids out. They're in their bed because Candice got all stirred up too early and wouldn't be quiet. So a time out was needed. I'm gonna lay back and rest for a few minutes. Now that things are done except for my nose irrigation.

41. Drove my blazer to town got Hunter to fix my prescription. He's so nice to me. The lady (can't remember her name) is too. She noticed my breathing hard and said I probably didn't feel like going to town – I said she was right. But I'm so congested and tired. I feel so sick. Like I need a tune-up. Again – we was gonna go to the movies and out to eat. That's off. I'm coughing too much to go see a movie. I'd still like to go get a haircut though. That just takes sitting there. As long as I could be quiet. God – please help me feel better, *please*!

42. Hey, Hey, Hey! I was coughing too much to go to the movies when Jimmy got home. I fell asleep on the bed for about 45 minutes. Then when I woke up he said lets go to Franklin and get a flashlight. His for work was torn up. So – we went. I got my Black purse! Just like the one at the mall! Only from Wal-Mart. It's suade and leather. Beautiful! Then we went to the mall, I saw Crystal there so I got my haircut. It's perfect! She's so good at it – always takes her time and does what I say I want. Then we got Jimmy's flashlight and back to Wal-Mart. For another purse. Just like the black one only camel colored. It was just to pretty to pass up. I had to have it plus they both had 29.96 price tags – only they rang up 19.96. What a deal. I was thrilled. They are so nice and so clean cut looking. Not worn out or cheap looking. I got the one on Sat. too. It's gorgeous and I love it. So I don't know when I'll swap them out. I'll rotate them maybe. I've been so congested

and coughing so hard that Jimmy said he's not sure if I'm getting better or not. I really had a hard time going to town. My mind was ok. It was my body. My legs are so weak. And my right leg is so sore in the hip that I can't sit indian style anymore. Using the bathroom is hard on me because it's low to the ground and hard.

Think I'll cook BBQ wings tomorrow that sounds good. I need to put some sauce over them. We went to Arby's for supper. Yeah! Yeah! Yeah! It was so good. I think I'll go get a bite of a leftover one now in fact. I moved in our regular room tonight. Less than ½ hour I'm up choking which concerns me. Since I was bleeding this morning my pluracy is acting up. I gotta go. I'm so sleepy. But first I need a drink of pepsi and bite of a sandwich.

43. I tried sleeping in our bed. I had to get up a few minutes after I fell asleep. Then I was up till 1 or so. Then I slept till 5 when Jimmy got up for work. I needed postral drainage. He gets so uptight when I ask him for that. He says it's such a waste of time. Because I'll be congested and coughing again in a couple hours. I told him that it helps me thru those couple of hours anyway. He said he had to go to work and he'd come by and use the buffer on me later. I said it's ok. I asked him to use that on me over the weekend and he didn't. Needless to say we aren't "close" anymore. I cannot breathe at all let alone be desirable. I feel like my life and health is slipping away. Before my own eyes. And it's effecting Jimmy's love for me. How could he really love and want me like I am? I cough so hard, so much, it really does make me ugly and

undesirable. The kids love me and stay so close as they can get to me. Jimmy tries sometimes. Like with the beautiful Valentines card and Roses. That shows he loves me. But who could blame him for being fed up with the rest of things day by day. I really probably should move in with Mom and Dad. Just so Jimmy can have the full carefree life he always says he wants. I only hear that he wants to date and so and so is a doll, it's not fair that this one or that one is "too cute" to be alone. And he bets she'd go out with him in a heartbeat he's so serious. He's not joking at all. I <u>never ever</u> felt so alone even when he's right beside me. Lord, Lord, this awful CF is ruining my marriage and everything else. We figure that a cruise that we wanted to go on will be out of the question. We talked to a travel agent last night. For a 3-4 day cruise on Carnival to the Bahamas will be like 600 per person (me and Jimmy). plus $80 each port fees and airfare to Ft. Lauderdale or Miami. Averaging out to like 1000 each. But Mom and Dad could go for 99. This is if we all four share a room too. Little, below deck room not to be rude or make Jimmy look bad; but I just thought of something. The other day during a little disagreement the subject of me wanting stuff came up. I wrote about it I think. Well, I mentioned that pizza Hut breadsticks would sure be good and lets get some (They always make one gain weight, but I didn't say that right then). Anyway, I was told no we didn't need any real quick. Now every time I ask Jimmy to take me out to eat he says we got food at home. If I say I'd like for him to pick me up something to eat while he's out and about. He says no cook whatever I asked for, here at home. Now that's ok – but why was he arguing that if I want something just say so 'cause he isn't going to ask if I need anything every time he goes out. Like I say up he says down. I say lets do that or whatever, he'll say no then later on argue that I never want to do anything as usual. I'm too sick to do anything. Like the cruise – he said yesterday that he really feels like I'm not better and he doesn't think I'd do too good on a cruise. Maybe not. I know they wouldn't be cheap plus mom kept telling *everyone* that we were going on one. Even Dr. Haynes. She asked me if I told him (one day while I was in the hospital) I said no I wasn't gonna mention it yet that I'd tell him later. First I wanted to get better and get home and healed up. .... Well, when he came in to see me one day and he got ready to leave she literally ran out of the room to catch him. I asked her the other day why. What did he say about my lungs or whatever. She said oh, nothing. That she was just telling him we were going on a cruise for a couple days in June. Now this was the last couple of days in June. When she was telling him and everyone else she could I was afraid she'd jinks it. I asked her not to but she kept on. Now the prices are so high and I'm still real sick so we doubt that I'll feel up to it. They may have alot to spend – we don't. Except for Jimmy's bass boat he says he wants and we'll have to build an addition on to the carport for it too. He says we can go and be on the lake all day – take the kids too. He wants it bad doesn't he? Last summer he said it was either too hot or too rainy on his days off to go boating if he had one. So who knows. I just thought of something else. Last night Jimmy said to me that he'd take his uniform shirts to the cleaners. They were the same ones he had cleaned last time. I said whatever, ok. Will you please take the pants too since they haven't been in a while and they need it. Especially for the professional crease. He said no, they aren't as cheap to clean – plus they can't be that much trouble to iron. I said I'd pay for it but he still didn't want to. So I might as well do the shirts too. No sense in just washing 3 pr. of pants by themselves. I can't figure some things out. At least he offered to do the shirts. One day I hope he reads this and realizes how much I love him and how he confuses me alot. I'm not sure if he really loves me or just tolerates me. Thats what I believe. The tolerating part. Oh yea he said put his pants in the dryer for a few minutes so I won't have to iron them. Wrong answer.

Well, the new flashlight Jimmy got yesterday is screwed up. It's his expensive THP flashlight too. It won't stay on. That figures. Everything we get we usually have to swap. We should just get 2 of everything everytime. Then keep the good one. It's crazy I know. We went grocery shopping after he got home. Then we went for a short walk to see where he's cleared more land. I had to pull my right blue jean leg up in order to get my right leg up as we walked. It's so weird. My legs are just not building up at all. No way. They are so weak. Still feel like they have weights on them. I went to see Casey. First time in a long time. He wanted to jump on me too. So I had to get out of his way fast. But Jimmy was being real sweet to me. I do love him. I wish he could understand how much. It's not just 'cause he puts up with me either. That's probably what he thinks. Not at all. I love him from the bottom of my heart. He can be so sweet and gentle and then so nasty and hurtful the next. But then so can I. I'm not as out of breath as I usually am after our walk. I thought it'd wear me out but I'm ok. A little short of breath. Like after I do housework. I'm so ready for Spring!! I got some really cool pens at Kroger. Papermate with a thick grip handle – so I can really hold it and write good. They were $3 but I had $1 off of 3. So it's a bargain. I'm sounding like I have TB or Bronchitis again. This shrill cough is bad – plus I'm short of breath still and hurting. So I need stuff for that. I'm sure it makes the shortness of breath worse – but if I'm spazzing out I gotta do something! The weather is nice in the day time. Mornings and nights are cold and that's when I spazz out. Anyway – I feel ok otherwise I guess.

44. I'm *NOT* believing this! It's Feb. 20th and I'm back in the hospital again!! I got sick real sick this morning and had a temp of 100.3 Teresa said go to the E.R. I did. As soon as Jimmy got in (early) – poor guy. He's upset and so am I. I can't write what Dr. Haynes said in the E.R. not yet. He asked if he could pray with us so we said sure. We all joined hands – he said a long prayer. Thanking God for the privaledge of taking care of me all the years etc. Getting to know me and Jimmy as a wonderful young couple etc. And asking him to give us the courage to face the future and what may happen unless a miracle comes along etc. Afterwards he was *crying*, Jimmy was crying and I was too. Dr. Haynes is so great. He's talking about maybe trying a respirator if I want to. He's got me on oxygen. A new shot for my breathing and morphine if the first shot don't work. Along with everything I always get. I had 7 sticks to get 1 IV and a blood test. So I'm

127

gonna get a central line put in my neck maybe tomorrow. Jimmy is really something else. He acts too tough. But he's not tough at all. He loves me alot. I know that. After our talk with Dr. Haynes, well he's been so huggy, kissy I love that. I'm scared. Really bad. I hate to have Mom and Dad come home early. But I need them so bad. I'm not sure what to do about things. I need to see what they think. The respirator business really scares me. It's to give the lungs rest. But a person can't talk, eat, or drink on one. So that's pretty bad. I'm shook up. Ok. This really could be the beginning of the end, ok. There I said it. Dr. Haynes said so. He's not saying that I'm really bad off. It's just my 3 trips here in 3 months. Nothing's helping nothing's clearing me up. What in the world will happen to my baby (Jimmy) or the kids if I stay here a long time? I can't stand being away from them. I love Jimmy so much. And the kids are my world too. I am just so upset. Please God. Hear my prayers, and Jimmy's and Dr. Haynes. Show us a miracle help me get better please! We lost Buddy today. Bless her heart. WE really loved her too.

45. It's nearly 2 A.M. and I'm up choking. As usual. Lord I hope Jimmy reaches Mom and Dad. I hate to ruin their vacation. But they won't come back if they don't want to. It's no biggy. Jimmy was going to stay the night but I told him to rest all he can. It'll be hard enough on him 'till Mom does get home perhaps they should talk to Dr. Haynes instead of me telling them what he said. We'll decide. Later – It's time for aerosole and a beating. The nurse just started to give me phenergan IV instead of IM. I stopped her

in time. They would have been trying to find a vein for sure if she'd had done that. I'm sleepy now. But respirtory will be around in a few minutes so I need to stay awake.

One day I need to see about getting my things at home in order. You know jewelry, purses, clothes, etc. Need to do that soon I guess. Mom I'm sending you a telepathic message. I need you! *BAD!*

Have I told you lately that I'm mad. Well I am. I want to go to Florida.

Ok – Here it is ok. Dr. Haynes says our bodies are like tents left out in the rain and weather they can only hold up for so long. Then they collapse. And CF patients can only go on for so long until our insides wear out. Our lungs get too tired to work and we just give away to a more perfect, peaceful place. And there are no pains or illness there. No sadness or anything bad. Get my drift? That's why I'm scared. I don't want to go any where but home to my husband and kids. They need me. I sure need them.

46 Nurse Rhonda took me to the caffeteria for a good breakfast. Then we came back to my room to eat. It was really good. And she gave me a stack of 3x5 cards to get other free meals with. She said get'em all there. It's better food. She's so nice. She said some things that make sense, because I was sort of upset. I coughed all night so the nurses want me to get some cough syrup to go in between codeine pills. Mom and Dad got the message at the condo.

Mom's awful upset. She was crying and carrying on so bad I said let me talk to Dad ok. She did. I told him what was what and so he knows. Now I don't know if they'll be coming home soon or not. Their week with the condo is up Sun. so they may come back sooner. What's gonna happen to Jimmy? OH GOD. I adore him. I love him with every ounce of my being. I couldn't live without him and I'm not sure if he'd be ok if I left him. He's as good as a mountin of Gold. 1 in a million. He tries so hard to be perfect at everything he does. The only problem there is – he doesn't have to try at all. I'm here in my room 670. He's at home I guess. I miss him. My kids, and my home. And the little things too. Gotta get my dolphin plate unwrapped and set up in the perfect spot. I got a shot of morphine for my chest/shortness of breath. It works better than the other stuff. But I don't like morphine. The oxygen really helps best. Gotta rest.

I'm back, my IV hurts a little bit. They are gonna put a central line in my neck. When this IV blows watch it blow at night. I'm so tired. I did not sleep last night. Jimmy said take a nap. I said no I'd rather be with him plus it might keep me from sleep.

47. Well, tonight I was let down again by Jimmy. No biggie to him. He decided he was going to the wake for Buddy and then tomorrow too. His Daddy said no he didn't need to leave me alone since I'm so sick. Jimmy said no problem if they needed him there he'd be there. I didn't know about his other plans for tonight. Todd was gonna come by and pick him up then drop him off again. Well,

I was trying to stay awake best I could. So when I got sick Jimmy, took off. Now anyway we we're watching TV and I dozed off. I was resting good with my chest. Then of course I was dreaming that the kids were running around the house I woke up. Startled because of the phone ringing loud. I just start sobbing. Well, I recognized my tears too. I could not help it but Jimmy got mad cause I cried. See I thought that I was home watching the kids playing. When I realized where I was I cried more before I could stop. Jimmy told Todd forget it he wouldn't be able to go afterall. Then he was sarcastic with me and he went to get me supper when he got ready. Wouldn't let me go this time. I went at lunch. It was fun. He's ashamed of me. I know. He can't help it. But I was talking to Julie about it while he was gone. And how much I missed my folks. I cried and she hugged me for 2 or 3 minutes. We cried and she said some real nice things about us and its the stress taking over. I'm so fed up. I told Jimmy to go ahead home – he'd either sit there going ugh-ugh-ugh for no good reason. Or watch out the door for Regina to strut by. Come sit by me and sleep! He got mad at me told me to be quiet and just go back to rest. I said no someone else would just call, plus any other thing. This morning sometime the lab called and said MRSA is growing out again! Isolation again! And I'll be here for no telling how long. Jimmy had to go call Debbie first off without asking me. I had reason. I wanted to see if that junk grew out for one, MRSA wanted to make sure they wasn't sick or sniffling in any way. In case they mentioned being up here for a visit. Cannot have that. I maybe go for the respiratory thing. To help me breathe easier. To help my breathing problem I don't know what to do I've gotta go to bed I'm sleepy. Maybe getting the other IV tomorrow this one is achy a little. Anyway – Jimmy left here mad. Because of the Todd calling business, waking me up. Excuse me, but if there's another time – if I get over this then I'm gonna be sure he tells his family to leave me alone. I'm fed up. His sergeant called me to tell me to make Jimmy use some of his sick days to be able to be with me more and take care of the dogs and house and him without being so tired. Well guess what. MRSA grew out again. Signs on the door – they called it in to Sheila the nurse before the reports came in! So NO ONE better come up. Sgt. Perry said he wanted to when he called awhile ago. I'm tired. I'm going to bed. Fed up! Something else to deal with Jimmy will probably get mad. I asked the nurse to put up a NO VISITORS sign. Except for Jimmy, Mom and Dad. That's all. I've gotta get some rest and it's the weekend some people I know will jump with chance to come visit like it's some party or something. Not.

48. Waiting on the people to put in the central line Jimmy came by for a bit. Went to get me lunch. Then we hung out awhile. He was remarking about the guys putting in the central line waiting 'till he needed to be elsewhere for Buddy's funeral. I told him to go on and go. I'd be ok. So he went. He doesn't even know where the place is. He wouldn't call and ask either. He's so indifferent sort of short and snappy one minute. When I said go on I'd suffer in silence. He said what's that supposed to mean? I said I'd make a horse face and not cry. Then he could make fun of me later. I wanted him here. But I *know* for a fact that

he'd be just like last night. Ticked off because he didn't get to go with Todd. He ignored me then went to sleep. When I woke him up he got mad. He might as well stay at the house. All he does is get smart with me unless he's hanging out with his family. Then he's ok. Sure this is no fun. But he doesn't have to come around if all he's gonna do is be nasty. Or girl watch. Truly, really, that's what he did all day yesterday. He'd watch the nurse he likes and make noises. Then when I shut the door he'd sit there and make remarks about stuff on TV. And me. I'm so give out. He's gotta stop this. Or I gotta get out. He remarked awhile ago that he could've bet 100 bucks that they'd wait till lunch time to put this dum central line in. Nevermind me. Nevermind what I'm gonna go thru. Do I ask too much? I don't really ask for anything. I just hope someone offers to be kind. But then kindness is everyones forté right? Some people are just different. Jimmy got irritated when I asked him to adjust the room temp in here a time or two the other day. He heard what doctor Haynes said the other day. He plainly heard him say to enjoy what time we have together and be grateful for the good times etc. Yet he refuses to let me in his thoughts. He's built a wall around his heart and he doesn't (and won't) let me in. He's always thought bad thoughts of me. All I do is love him. Just like he is – faults and all. This other girl business had better stop! I'm fed up to my eyes with it. He won't hush. It's all I hear about. Well, he's been saying for me to go so he can get a newer model. He may say he's joking. He's not though and after what Dr. Haynes said Thurs. he'll get his wish. We aren't sure how long. But he'll get his way. He always does doesn't he? I always get the shaft. Thanks alot! As for last night I slept some off and on. I couldn't get my aerosole till late. Then I had IV's then I coughed so it was like that off and on. My IV had an ocllusion 4 times. I wacked it good on the table this morning. Not meaning to. God – I miss Mom and Dad! What I'd give to see them walk thru that door! But they're in Florida. Wish I was too. This place ain't so bad. I'm getting used to it. It sure ain't home. But the nurses are so nice. Last night while Jimmy went for my supper I just couldn't take it anymore. Julie my nice nurse who wants to give me an AKC German Shepherd) came in like every 10 minutes or so to see if I was ok all day long – came in – I couldn't help myself. Jimmy had smarted off to me again. I started to cry. She did too. She gave me a hug. Said what can I do. Please just tell me. I said just hug me a minute ok. She did. She talked to me and I calmed down. I love Jimmy. But he's not taking things to well. He's trying to push me away so much one minute then reaching out to me when I need him. It's too confusing. Like today. I really need him. I'm scared ok. Who wouldn't be. Where's he at? Not with me. I wish to God Mom and Dad would walk in. I need them. My heart aches for them to be here. I don't expect Jimmy to be. He's fed up. He's worn out. And he's ready for something new. He'll be there for Donna. She's got people there. I don't. I told him to go. I knew he'd never let me forget it otherwise. I'm always lost. Always the awful uncaring person. Selfish etc... that's what he says. Oh yea. That's why I let myself go thru things on my own. It's never appreciated. Never acknowledged. Not by him. His dad said he should be here. Jimmy said – what's Donna want? That's what I'll do. Excuse me. I love Donna also. Really.

But, well never mind. When he left here last night he *was* mad. Today he says no he wasn't. Well, I saw different. I think I'll have to go live with Mom and Dad. When I told Dr. Miller I needed this oxygen when I went home he said sure that can be arranged. Jimmy grunted and made that "oh no" face. Meaning he'd be embarrassed who cares I need to breathe! I hear them out by my door. Don't know who it is. I'm sleepy. I'm scared. I want to run! I want to scream, yell, slap something I want my *Mom*. Dad makes me feel so safe I want him to hug me. I feel so scared lately. So lonely. Why? Me and Jimmy aren't in sync any more. I know it's over with us. The stuff he's done for me lately has been sweet and nice. But why do I still feel so lonely. When I really need him he's either there and being sort of cocky (like get over it already) or he's not even there. I'm going nuts. Every time I see a shadow by my door. If they'd take me down stairs I'd feel better. I think. Maybe my nurse Carol will be able to stay here with me. Let ya know later how it goes. Gotta rest now. I'm too sleepy. I miss the way I used to feel and look. Now I'm all boney. I disgust Jimmy I know it. I disgust myself. He said to call him when I get my thing done. I'm not though. If he was worried enough he could've stayed. He didn't so I'm not gonna go outta my way. Just had to get a shot of phenergan too. I think I'm gonna hurl my lunch. Why can't I see straight? My mind wanders alot. I wonder if Jimmy ever loved me. Really. Maybe. Maybe not. I'm thinking alot. Not alot of love I'm thinking alot of things. My IV hurts! It's about to beep too. I'm sleepy. I was hesitant to call for phenergan because of that. But I had to. Now I know

I look weird. I feel a headache coming on. I'm gonna need a chest pain shot too.

49. Got it! The Central. Bled all over and had to go for it twice. Small veins even in my chest and neck. But I got 4 mgs of morphine. I'm so out of it when I cough I feel it. On my collar bone. Got some (looks like just 2 on outside) stitches to hold tube in place. Aches now like if someone punched me in the shoulder. Jimmy came in 'bout ½ hour afterwards. Looked at it and me. I think he really wanted me to call him. But I can't call anyone. I'm so doped up wish I had the old IV out of my hand. It hurts. But Carol is busy I guess.

50. MOM and DAD ARE HOME. THANK THE LORD!

51. Jimmy just left. I told him to go now. I'm fed up. He's not gonna stand in my room and ball me out every single day. The ones I can count on are back. So I'll be ok. He was smarting off to me since he got here. I'm wheezing so I should take my beatings. I am. I just skipped the one about an hour after my central line was in. It feels like surgery. My whole surgery hurts! Then he yells at me for something else. I can't remember now. But he got mad because I ran out of t.p. Had to use my roll I brought. It's half gone. I needed to go! So I asked him to ask for a roll for me. Well he did about an hour ago. Not quite but close to. It's still not here. I used my own. But he smarts off that I should just ask for it. Only I did. The cleaning lady said ok. But she didn't put any there! What can I do about it. I was

having a catheter put in so I couldn't watch her to see if she brought any in. No big deal. But he starts this hoarding stuff business. Just use what I have ---- I shouldn't worry so much ---- I'm so disgusted with him and his behavior. It's one thing to come up here to be helpful. But not to start a fight! His remarks are not necessary or wanted. He found out one thing. I'm congested because I was getting 60 mg. codeines every 4 hr. Can you imagine? The nurses messed up. So – he smarts off again. Why did I take 'em? As for the t.p. He said just ask for some. I can't get the people to do anything too fast. I'd really be in a mess if I did. I mean – he sees how they are himself. Yet, things are always my fault. He's so darn mad at me for everything. Whether it's my fault or not. And I'm tired of it. He needs help. Sometime soon. He's making me so miserable. Over t.p. and codeine. What a deal. Why doesn't he love me for me. I didn't ask for this. He could choose to help me not cause me to be upset. And definately *not* make me throw him out which is what I did. I told him to get the – out of my room now I did not need to be yelled at or told off. He left. The guys got a giant chip on his shoulder and I'm tired of being blamed for it. Nice Valentine card and roses. Nice Valentine card verse. Where'd that come from anyway. Like he means it. Oh sure. He acts it. One day I hope he realizes how snotty he has been. One day he'll see that I'm not this dumb jerk he acts like I am. One day he'll be sorry. He can keep his butt home from now on if he wants. I don't care. He hates being here as much as I do. Only I'm supposed to sit back, enjoy it. And ask if I want anything. I can ask – but I won't get it. I waited over 6 hours to get an old IV pulled. Over an hour for t.p.

You get the idea. Well, the nurse just came in to unhook my IV. Said the "server" whoever that is will give me tp. I said ok thankfully she brought me some just now. 1 hour 15 minutes plus an argument. Hope it's lined with gold! What's wrong with this world anyway. What's wrong with me. Why does Jimmy hate me so much? I can't help what's happening to me. Dr. Haynes said in his prayer to please help Jimmy with his grief and help us both to be strong. Help me cope with what's going on, help me help Jimmy. That sure sounds like a lot to ask. So far all I feel is hatred from Jimmy and anger. He cannot stand to be near me now. When I really need him to love me and be understanding. He backs out on me. It hurts me. Knowing how most of it is not my fault at all. And I have to deal with *all* of it and him not being nasty. I remember now what he got testy about. He mentioned the isolation/no visitors. (I added that) the names who was by me last time. Only 3 Mom, Dad and of course Jimmy. Well, he tells his Dad and them Oh I'm pretty sure it doesn't mean family. Dah – for god's sake wake up – I don't need any more germs at all. None. And goodness knows his family has been around lots and lots of people the past few days. I don't need any more chances of germs than I'm getting in here. He goes and tells everyone that and before you know it I'll have something else for him to gripe about. I'm the one with no immune system. I'm the one that's, well, you know. Can't he see what's happening? Doesn't he care or what? So what if I bring t.p. here. It's a good thing I did. So what if I skip a beating after a surgical procedure? So what. That's all little dumb things. Not worth the trouble. Not worth going to bed mad over. I'm right. He doesn't care. He doesn't. It's not fear or anything. It's pure old dislike for me. I still love him. I can't blame him – I wouldn't love me either. I'm tired 'till later.

52. Early 23rd. Talked to Peggy last night about Jimmy. She said she has a feeling she understands his problem. She's pretty sure he's going thru the grief stage just watching me. That's why he's so sweet and nice one minute and upset and cranky the next. She said Dr. Haynes would be the best one to talk to him alone about it. Now we gotta get them together somehow. Huh?/Yeah! Mom and Dad are home. Gonna come up and see me soon. Yeah!

53. Sun. A.M. I'm hungry! Slept all night. Wish I could talk to Jimmy. I miss him. I love him. And he could go get me some food too. That would be nice. But he never comes up early. So I guess I'll just have to wait on the rotten breakfast I'll probably get. I want biscuits and gravy. Those from downstairs the other day were so good. I'm still tired I'm coughing alot – so that's why. I'm feeling clearer today. Because I've taken less codeine. I could use one now actually. And a percocet too. I've got a headache. I can't stand arguing with Jimmy. He just hovers around and finds things to be upset about. Or he does other things that make me nervous. Then he'll say be calm – I usually am. Except now. I am hungry.

54. I'm so happy today. Jimmy came in early to see me. He brought me stuff and he was in a good mood. Later he went and got me breakfast and we ate together. Then later after Mom and Dad came in Jimmy went shopping

for me. I got new sleepshirts and Kleenex and it was so sweet of him. I needed shirts with a lower front for my catheter to be easily accessible. He got me 2 really cute ones! Mom and Dad brought me turtles, a dolphin T-shirt, a porcelain clown doll all kinds of goodies. Then Sgt. Perry and his wife came by and brought me an angel bag full of Avon things and you'll never guess what? $50 for gas and food money. Wasn't that great of him. His wife is really sweet too. We had to explain what's going on (we meaning me and mom). The guys were out. So we told Sgt. Perry I wanted to be sure that he looks after Jimmy and takes him under his wing if he needs it. You know what I mean I hate to share all stuff with people but he needs to know so he'll just be "in the know". But I pray I'll be ok for months maybe years to come. I've got to try. For Jimmy and the kids and everyone else too. We've managed to get a few things out in the open. I drank a whole carton of that nutritious stuff. So I made everyone happy and be proud of me. It's getting later after 1. Don't ask. Meds. were late, aerosole was later. Then they ran the big IV bag in so now I'm waiting on it I've got the TV on we watched that new show tonight – King of the Hill. It's great. Funny and different. I'd like to see it more. Man I've gotta get some sleep. It's getting warm in here.

55. Man. Less than 3 hrs. sleep. I'll be tired today. I asked the nurse about my sputtum sample last night. He said all kinds of things were growing out of it. But pseutiomosas was sure enough there. After all the anti-biotics I've had lately too. Wonder what Dr. Haynes will say we could try

some of the old meds even if they effect my ears. What does it matter anyway. If these aren't helping you know we need to do something.

56. NO WAY – CANNOT BELIEVE THIS, VANKOMYACIN AGAIN! GOT MRSA BACTERIA BAD! Pseudomon BAD! What's going on here? Why did that Ranky Vank have to come back in the picture? Don't like it. Don't want it either.

57. Rough day – Coughed alot. Real icky stuff too. Getting alot up. Gonna get the sinus surgery done next Mon. if my lungs can handle it. Dr. Courey said he'd try knocking me out "if" Dr. Haynes says ok. Otherwise it'll be a "local". The surgery takes 2 hours. No black eyes or big swelling. Just discomfort and feeling bad for a couple weeks. Today has been crazy. The nose doctor said something about me going home next Tuesday. That's really weird - 'cause Dr. Haynes hasn't even mentioned it to me. Especially with me having all this icky infection in my lungs and the MRSA showing up again. Over growing in the lab. One ½ weeks of stuff won't help that. We'll see tomorrow what Dr. Haynes says. Right now I'm so congested it's awful. Peggy wants me to talk to another patient here. One that has a bad lung problem too. She carries on pretty good and there is no way I'm gonna do that. I'm not going. Can't do whatever they say. I'm not getting with her while I'm so sick. I'm finally getting some help and hope. So I don't need anymore germs plus my Dr. says no unexpected guest. I'm sleepy and just frustrated <-- WHATEVER! (next day) Hey, I'm going to get to go to the deli and get

breakfast with my friend Rhonda. So I'll at least get a doughnut and big ole cup of grapejuice plus I'm gonna see about a BLT and home fries. Sounds good I know! EXTRA Bacon. I asked Mom about Aunt Shirley. She changed the subject or I did one. 'Cause she didn't say how she is. I don't remember. My baby called me last night. I talked to him awhile (heard'em say (Trooper Pitts) over the radio. I was so excited. He was riding with the Sgt. I told him what Dr. Courey said. He said he thought he was mixed up too.

58. Ok – got it down now. Saw Dr. Haynes. I am gonna have the sinus surgery. Be knocked out "general" because it's only for 2 hours or so. That's too long for a "local" he said. Well, this type of surgery, it's gonna be a week long stay like Dr. Courey said. Only I was right – there was no talk of me going home on Tues. Don't know where he got that anyway. I'm so sleepy. I got up early for breakfast and now I'm tired. Dad came up here today to be with me while Mom stayed with Lee in Dickson. She had a DNC. Anyway – this "Vank" is making me nauseated and the vertigo is back again. It's a smaller dose but it's still strong. I've only had 2 bags and already have side effects. Gotta rest now. I'm exhausted. Almost aresole time though. Gee wiz. No rest at all. And you know what else? At *least* two more weeks of this. Maybe longer. We have no idea. But not until I get rid of this infection.

59. Today I felt pretty good when I got up. As the day went on I got real congested. I don't know why really. I've been coughing and clearing out. But respiratory has been

screwing up aeresol times – plus nutra-shake's. Bet that is it. It's a dairy product! I'll skip today then try it again. Dad stayed here and kept me company 'till Lee's thing was done. Then him and Mom came back. Jimmy showed up and stayed late. I couldn't stay awake. Phenergan made me so sleepy. Oh and he tucked me in and kissed me so sweet before he left. I couldn't eat my supper he got me. I tried.

60. Haven't felt good today. Too congested. Found out that it's probably nutrashakes. So I'll quit drinking them. Just found out that the throat and nose can cause you to have congested sounds if the sinuses are infected – so this surgery should "please" help. I'm still scared.

61. Got a temp. 100.2. Don't think this stuff's working. Maybe we should try something else? (Dr. Haynes said it's working.) 2-27

62. Man, what a day yesterday. Migraine City. Bad one too. Every partical of skin, every tiny hair on my body ached and hurt. It was awful and I was sick at my stomach and all that.

63. Been sleeping thru the nights! I get up with my oxygen under my arm alot. My temp is 99. today. Still have no idea about my surgery. They just sent the forms to be signed like it was today. I'm starting to get irritated here. A week without my kids is driving me nuts. I want my babies. I miss being home too. I want Jimmy to snuggle up with me on the couch and watch a movie. So I can lay

my head on his shoulder and go to sleep. Of course the kids would be there too. All of us together. Oh gee whiz – my eyes is hurting again. My migraine is coming back. It's gotta be a combination of surgery and everything else combined. Please make this headache go away. I washed my hair again because yesterday it got all messed up by my being in bed sleeping all day. It looked awful. The way I felt. I should write Debbie and Aunt Shirley. But I don't feel like it. I'm gonna rest. Maybe it'll be a good day. I miss Jimmy.

64. I'm so mad. My diabetes is acting up now. They're sticking my finger and giving me insulin. Like I don't have enough to worry about. My insulin shots are givin in my stomach. Dr. Haynes ordered it 4 times a day. Why I'll never know. Well yea I do. My sugar was 550 then 386 then 377. My medicine is being mixed in D5W. (Sugar water!) I mentioned it and was told it's not enough to hurt. Oh sure, it's not their belly being givin insulin shots huh. I'm tired. But I'm starting to get mad. That Dr. Courey won't tell me anything about my nose surgery. He still hasn't been around. I'm sleepy.

65. Woke up at 6 today. Got my finger stuck and an insulin shot within the first 5 minutes. I wonder if they'll do all this Mon or Tues? I'll be out of it if it does or if they do.

66. Since I'm going under a "general" I'll write down a few things. I'm hoping for the best, but one never knows. The page will be stuck in here. My right arm is numb. It's storming out bad.

67. I'm fed up! TOTALLY FED UP! I try so hard to be happy and easy going but I have my limits! Jimmy came back from getting my lunch – mad – because he had so much to carry. He's mouthing off to me and frowning. I ask what's wrong and he snaps at me. I'm so tired of it too. It's not easy being here and I can't leave the room. Like the other day when I went to see Dr. Courey and Jimmy said he'd carry the oxygen tank. All he did was gripe about it and say leave it next time and he wouldn't want to fool with it anymore ---- No one asked him to carry it. He said he would now he's mouthing off to me and saying it's my meds. Not him. Wrong. He's not listening to himself. He's not acting nice and I don't appreciate it. Now I told him to leave and go on wherever he was going and leave me alone. So he did. He's been gone about 6 hours so far. He's saying one thing and doing another. Like he says 1 minute that he's gonna work Monday (my surgery day) then when I mention him working he yells that he's taking the day off and I knew that! Then he'll say something else another time. So I don't know what he's gonna do. I mention that there's no reason anyone has to wait on me for my surgery and he snaps that his "sister" or "his" friends "Roger and Debbie" can come and sit if they want. No reason for that at all. He doesn't even have to be here as far as I am concerned. I was just told by Mom that I have a home to go to if I want to move home that's good to know. I feel like Jimmy is at his wits end. I know I am. I'm not shutting him out – he did me first. I'm just tired of everything. I walked in place for at least 15 minutes and still had to have insulin. I couldn't believe it. Insulin screws me up like steroids do. I don't have a choice though. I had spasms and needed some

more morphine. I hope Dr. Haynes doesn't care. I needed something fast. Whatever. He's back. As I'm getting my morphine. He doesn't like for me to get that. But if I have to I have to. I'm tired. The anesthesiologist came in. He says I'll be dopey and all that like with my gallbladder. Then they'll do the respirator and surgery part. Then take me off the respirator and hopefully I'll do ok. If not then they'll knock me out more and put it back in. We hope it goes ok. From the minute they pull the tube. I'm really scared. If I wake up and it's in I'm supposed to just relax. But I'd freak out for sure.

68. 3/1. Still upset. Jimmy went home. I'm glad. I want to be alone. Things with us aren't right. Too many secrets, too much confusion. Jimmy went to Centerville the other day. Never said anything about it to me. I get a card saying how glad they are to hear I'm feeling so much better from the Nashs'). I'm not. Then Jimmy gets mad at me when I asked him about it. Like how they knew I am sick. And why do they think I'm better? He got mad at me and yelled because I was asking too many questions. Then last night he left here early because it was storming outside and he needed to check on the dogs. He called Becky from the cell phone (instead of here) and went to her house. That's ok. That's good. But he could've called me to let me know he got home and the kids were ok. At least let me talk to them a minute! But NO! He won't even tell me how they are if I ask. He smarts off that they're fine quit worrying. I'm not worried – I just want to see how my babies are. Another thing he does is he'll get me upset by snapping at me then he'll tell me to hush

and just relax. Or lay back and take a nap and be quiet etc... I can't take this stress. He didn't even ask me about my surgery after I said the anesthesiologist was in here. He just acted like it was no big deal. It's not – at least not to him. And he said he was at his Dad's all day and his Dad wasn't home. Donna and Todd was. See – whenever I come in here he seems to enjoy going to his family's and all that. It's what he wants to do. And that's ok with me. He needs this support. But he really is hard on me. He acts weird towards me. Like he doesn't want to be near me. Like I'm poison. I may not go home with him. At least not to stay. We'll see if I come off the respirator on Mon. and when I go home.

69. It's the night before my surgery. I'm scared. Alots going on in my mind. I'm irritable. I'm trying not to show it though. Jimmy's gone out to eat. Mom and Dad are gone to get me supper. Every little thing makes me jump. My sugar was 140 yeah! No insulin right now. My head aches so bad. And not to mention my ribs. I wonder how I'll do off of oxygen when I go home?

70. My ribs ache and so does my bones. I'm so sore I can barely move. If I get to go home I think I'll be able to get around but I probably will need some help for awhile. Mom said she might come over and help cook for a couple days at a time. I'll see what happens. Dr. Courey still hasn't came to see me yet. Belinda said that I'm such a joy to have as a patient. She said everyone on the floor just loves me. I'm always cheerful and easy going. I said thanks. And I wonder if Jimmy felt the same way. I promise.

I'm no different here than I am at home. Really. Yet I hear different things at home. Jimmy went to eat a long time ago. I guess he's visiting his Dad and Donna. Who knows. Mom and Dad left too. So I'm alone, and I started coughing up blood too. My head hurts. I'm starting to get worried about tomorrow. I have such high hopes that I'll be able to breathe easier and maybe smell and taste too. I pray I'll be able to. And I pray I get off the respirator too. That really has me worried. I'm scared to be put to sleep. Jimmy said Donna and Lynn want to come by around 4 to see me. Only I'll still be in surgery. I wish and hope they can all sit here and wait together. Jimmy needs someone and after all – we are all family. Not friends or mere acquaintance. I don't want just anybody waiting around because I just don't. I don't need a reason!

71. I got up around 4'ish so sweaty that I had to change clothes. My sugar levels were ok. 84. That's why I was sweating. And hungry! I wanted to snack. Thought I could but it's jello and juice, yippee! Jimmy stayed late last night. He was real sweet. I guess he had some things to work in his mind. We said last night that we're scared. But he said it'd be ok.

72. Man I'm nervous. I want to get out of here. I'm so shaky and I just spilled apple juice all over. I was gonna go shower but I'm waiting on Dr. Haynes. Respiratory hasn't been in yet. I got up too early that's what's going on. I'm tired. I put a sign on the door so people wouldn't knock so loud. They probably won't pay it any attention. I nearly jump out of bed when they knock on the door. It bounces off

the wall – like I'm doing myself (bouncing off the walls). I see people cooking on TV. Noodles and parmesan cheese. You know, that sounds and looks good. Just plain noodles with some butter and sprinkle with cheese, lemon pepper and salt. That and some chicken maybe. I think I need to go home and fix some myself. Actually, I think I need a nap! But I have stuff going on.

73. 3/5. Had the surgery. Man I'm sore! My nose is swollen and stuffy. But I made it. The operation was delayed an hour or so, and I was just hanging around waiting (knocked out of course). I got back in my room after 8 o'clock. But it's been 2 days and I'm still sore. Dr. Courey made me squirt water in my nose and try to blow my nose! Ouch. He left 2 tubes in my nose too. Gotta go Mon. and get them taken out. Today Jimmy showed out in front of Mom. Over lunch. He thought I was gonna make a scene over what lunch I had. When all I "was" gonna say was I had to wait to eat until they stuck my finger to check sugar levels. Well, he got mad and smarted off if I didn't like what I got to get Mom and Dad to go get me something else. Only he really said it hateful. Mom looked so surprised. She's never heard him smart off to me like that. Afterwards she said she had no idea Jimmy could be so rude to me. It was all she could do to hold back about me being sick and how he shouldn't be hateful to me. I was really hurt by Jimmy. I had seen a different side to him the day of my surgery. He was sweet and kind. And scared. He kept hugging me and kissing me on the top of my head a bunch of times. Then the next day he got me a get well card from the kids and put their paw

prints by their names. *So* cute. Then today he got mad at me for absolutely no reason. My sugar levels are high too. We don't know why. I'm not eating alot or drinking many juices. Just strawberry kiwi juice, which is supposed to be diet. Oh well, I may get to go home this weekend. Maybe. Dr. Haynes cut down on my steroids today and I feel it. We'll have to wait and see. I'm real upset over this nasty mouth business though. I'm hurt and upset. I just ate an Arby's roast beef for a snack. It's 10 o'clock. Sort of late for a big snack but if I didn't eat it I'd feel bad. 'Cause Jimmy got'em for me. So much is going on in my mind. I've got things to be yanked out and all that – I'm scared it's gonna hurt too. (My chest IV and 2 tubes in my nose). I may wait 'till Mon. to go home. That's what Mom and Dad say to do. But that's a whole weekend in here again. They're so boring! I'm just so darn upset. How could Jimmy be so mean to me? Why? What did I do? He was mad at me for no particular reason as usual I don't know what to do. I may have to do insulin at home too Lord I hope not. I've got all this to deal with, I've got laryngitis as usual, and certain people keep coming here to my room bugging me so I had to turn my phone off. Then they called the nurses station to send messages! I'm, like, leave me alone. Get the message already. It's like the old guy that sells the paper here. Everyday he'll knock real loud and say wanna buy a paper. I say no. He doesn't pay attention to the quiet, do not disturb etc....signs on the door. And he'll wake you up all the time. And scare you when he knocks real loud. I'm ready to get out of here. But physically I'm not so sure about.

74. Today I am seeing double. My head hurts and I can't breathe good. I went 11 hours without pain medicine. I asked for a percocet 2 hours (little less really) ago and never got it so I called for morphine still can.

75. I go home tomorrow. My head hurts but I'm better. My nose is clearing up. My swelling's going down. Jimmy didn't come by. Hope he isn't mad or being rude. After yesterday I'm scared he's mad. But I didn't do anything he did. He better not have went to see his Mom and not me or I'll be mad. See this family business is causing problems again. But I'm not getting in the middle of it. I hope I get alone ok from all this sickness. I hope I can breathe at home too. I'm scared to have this catheter pulled out tomorrow. And my nose tubes Monday too! My right arm hurts now. Where I've had all the shots in. My feet are swollen and I'm sore all over. Mom wants me to finish my book. Well, add on to it. Everybody does. I don't know if I will or not. I may add some to it. But it'll be awhile. I just wanna get home and relax. I pray me and Jimmy are "ok" after this. He was so nice. I haven't saw him very much though. He pretty much left things up to Mom and Dad and he's done the taken care of business at home job! That's hard enough. My nose is real sore. I just bumped it with my oxygen mask. I've gotten a bunch of clots out of it today. I know it's gross sounding – but I did. And I can breathe easier too. I got the coolest pill book from Mom and Dad. It's a nurses type book. *Easy* to look up stuff. I love it. But it was way too expensive ($30.00). Dr. Haynes gave me a new kind of pain pill and I looked it up. It's in there! Today is Mom's birthday

and she spent it here with me in this place. That's no fun. She said she wanted to be here. My family's type of love is different than Jimmy's. He shows his love so differently. I wonder if I'll need to use the spare room or if I'll be able to sleep good and not bother Jimmy. We'll see. Oh yea – that nurse that made me crazy the other night, we told another one about her. Word got back to the first one and she actually asked me about why I complained on her and blah, blah, blah. That was weird. I just said I was doped from surgery and left it at that. But she was and is a tough type to deal with.

76. Woke up early. Dr. Haynes said he'd be here before 6. It's after 7 and he's not showed up yet! Jimmy is supposed to come and get me to go home. Now what'll happen. I can't breathe thru my nose today. I'm so anxious about going home and this catheter being pulled that I'm like a giant panic attack. If I get to go home today it'll be a miracle.

77. Cannot believe it but they say Dr. Haynes forgot to leave my discharge orders! He was at the end of the hall Thurs. night and did a person there's discharges. He said he'd be by my room Fri. before 6 A.M. He never showed. So we had to wait and wait for him to answer his page. He never did. Teresa let me go though. She took charge. The catheter removal was awful. It hurt; which I knew it would. So I get some morphine before they took it out. Sat. will be my first full day out of the hospital. It's dreary out so far. Maybe it'll cheer up out and I will too. I need to get a glucose monitor and some strips. I am not

looking forward to sticking my fingers all the time. And the thought of taking insulin makes me nuts. Jimmy is antsy. He's got 4 days off and he can't think of what to do first. He's been trying to put a bed cover on his truck that he had ordered. But he can't get it to do right. I can't figure it out either. I'm gonna order some cards and stuff from current. Oh yea – my nose is still *SORE* and bleeding and my face is still really swollen. I'm miserable after I go to sleep and wake up – I have a tough time breathing. Monday I should be able to.

78. I'm so fed up. My body is changing before my eyes and I can't control it. My ankles and knees are all swollen for no reason. After we went to the drugstore and grocery stores I took off my shoes and socks. There they were like double their size. I am so worried somethings wrong. What'll I do now? I'm gonna keep them elevated and maybe soak them. But first thing Jimmy says to me when he saw them is "I've had about all of this I can handle". I'm like, Thanks alot. Here I am totally freaked out and he says that's all he can take! What about me? What can I do? I know he wants out – to be free of the worries and medicines etc... But I can't turn off love like that. Either you really love someone and hang on with them or else you're outta there. Looks like he wants outta here. Only this is his house. Comes down to the same thing. Me leaving. I don't want this to be like it is. I love him. I hoped my sinus surgery would be a big help. He isn't even waiting for the results of that before he gives up hope. He *always gripes*. All the way home from the hospital. All afternoon and then

all day today. That's what he does. Gripes and carries on about what he could be or should be doing if I could. But I can't. And he never lets up about it. He does not like me at all. He really tries to hide it but he can't. It comes out in so many ways. I'm alone in this fight. So alone and scared. I just wish it could be different. I really wish we could pull together instead of apart when I need him the most. Maybe he's scared. Maybe he loves me. But maybe he doesn't and just can't say it. His actions show it. So I guess I'll move out when Mom and Dad get central heat and air. I haven't got a choice anymore. I'm so hurt and confused. I'm so mad. My face is swelled. My body is bruised and ugly. Now my feet are fat. Please God – give me a break! I'm fed up! I'm ready to be normal and be able to enjoy life a little. Just a little that's all. I deserve it! I do! Well I just got back from getting a glucose monitor. Hunter fixed me up with one and didn't charge me. He gave me strips for it (100) and lancets too. Sugar is 187. Not bad at all for me after a big supper, and dessert. Plus a banana.

79. The swelling in my ankles is going down. This morning they look more normal. I'm gonna leave them up most of the time today. Candice woke me up early crying. She wants to be close to me. So does peaches. In fact they both get all over me and give me sugar kisses often. Only had my nose bumped twice! Ouch! Jimmy is sleeping alot. He said he's tired. It's part boredom too. I think. He wanted to rent a movie last night. Glad he didn't 'cause he fell asleep after 10 o'clock. My muscles ache in my legs. I walk weird, but I'm going to rub them with some stuff and see

if it helps. We were going to see a movie and go out to eat at Uncle Bud's today. I wonder if we'll go?

80. We went to eat and see Vegas Vacation. Good food/Good movie. Now it's late but I can't go to sleep. I'm scared of tomorrow. Don't know about this tube business. I'm scared. Plus my sugar is high. For no reason. I don't want Dr. Haynes to make an issue outta it.

81. 3/12. Skipped some days. I'm feeling better. Still not real good. Sinus headaches and stiff legs. Short of breath too. But I'm better. Got the tube out of my nose on Mon. and it wasn't painful. But he washed out my sinuses all the way up behind my eyes!) and the suction from that hurt alot. I was really aching when we got there. I can breathe thru my nose real good but of course it's still real sore and swollen. Will be for awhile. Julie called to see how I'm doing that was real nice of her. I told her about my feet swelling and my sugar being high. I think that Bactrim is making my sugar high. It hurts my stomach so bad. And that's what effects the sugar levels - the stomach. All I know is that since I started it my sugar has been higher at night after I take my doses for the day. It screws my body up. But it's for the MRSA staph. I hope it gets rid of it 'cause I'm tired of having that. I want to feel good again. It's almost Spring! I want to enjoy it.

82. Ick! Today's our anniversary and Jimmy's working nights! It's gotten cold and gloomy out too. But I'm feeling pretty good. We went out to eat at KFC's for lunch. My nose is sore on the right side. I'm afraid it could be infected. I sure

hope not! They didn't give me enough antibiotic to flush it with though. They're crazy thinking about 3 inches of liquid anti-biotic will be enough to use several times a day in the bulb syringe for 14 days! I'm only supposed to use it twice a day though. Anyway I'm almost out and it hasn't been a week yet. Gotta talk to Dr. Courey about it Monday. Me and Jimmy have gone out to eat and see a movie 3 times this week! It's been fun. We've saw Vegas Vacation, Dante's Peak, and Howard Stern's private parts movies. All good. Now it's Friday our anniversary and nothings on TV. Jimmy slept all afternoon and I'm trying to get rid of a sinus headache. Yesterday he worked days. Sgt. Perry got me a beautiful stain glass Dolphin for the kitchen window. It's so pretty too. Now all we need is some sunshine to show it off. Lee sent us an anniversary card (Mom and Dad did too). But Lee didn't write in it or sign it "love". Nothing. Just their names. I wonder if she's mad at me. Because of the hospital situation. Isolation. She couldn't come and visit. Not like she needed too anyway she had her own stuff going on to rest up from. But anyway – I wonder why people ignore others until something goes on then all of a sudden take notice? Then ignore you again? Doesn't make sense. But if we'd have allowed her and John and Jen in then how would that look for the others who wanted to visit and couldn't? Not like isolation that's for sure. If someone gets ticked off over that then they aren't very nice. I wish she'd have written a few lines to me, really though.

83. Well, I go see Dr. Courey tomorrow. My nose is sore today and I have a bad headache too. We slept late so that could

be the reason for the headache. I really hope my nose isn't infected. The anti-biotic they gave me wasn't enough to last a whole week; but I don't know if it would have helped the soreness. I hope Dr. Courey doesn't get ugly about it. He has a strange way about him. Dr. Haynes has spoiled me that way. He's so nice to me.

84. Jimmy talked to his Dad today. We may go to Lynn and Donna's next week for steak! As long as things are going ok. I hope to goodness I stay healthy. I'm half scared to do anything or make plans for stuff. I need to talk to Donna though. Lynn too. I've missed them. I think I need a pep talk. Just to pump up my determination, you know? They have faith in me (even when I don't!). Ole Todd starts his 3rd week of Trooper school. He's doing ok in it. I worry about him and hope they don't bug him too much. He is a Pitts afterall and Lynn says he has enemies in high places. So they could make school tough for Todd. That school is hard enough. I'm so proud Jimmy got thru it when he did. Oh yea – Jimmy gets to take charge of the kids and the Big Circus next Sat. again. I wish I could go. But no way – not a million kids. And I'd have to chaperon and ride a school bus too. No thanks!

85. Went to see Dr. Courey. You wouldn't believe the clots he got out of my sinuses. I'm not joking. It's no wonder that my right side of my nose hurts. That whole side was blocked by clots. He said my nose shouldn't be bleeding anymore. But it is. I'm supposed to go see him "again" next week. Also the nurse said I'm gonna have to use the

anti-biotic irrigation for at least 6 months. It was supposed to be only a couple of weeks. That's the way it goes. More meds. I'm not feeling so good. My head hurts. On the way home it began to rain and we hydro-planed the Blazer into a big car. My poor Blazer! It's all messed up. We have to see about getting it fixed and all that tomorrow. It's a miracle we weren't hurt. Thank God we are ok. Oh yea – I got a new aerosole pump. It's real nice and quiet. It makes treatments go faster. I like it.

86. Oh Lord what a day. We went shopping in Franklin. Got a new blow dryer, beautiful leather boots for 6 bucks on clearance at Target! Alot of bargains to be had and we got 'em. I also got my Current order. Beautiful cards! Then to top it off a guy from NFL Alumni called me Ken Avery. He played for the Bengels, Giants and some other team. He's gonna get me an autograph picture of Dan Marino. And Dan's on a cruise this week. (I'm not kidding about this!!) But when he gets back Ken's gonna see if he will call me! Dan Marino! I'm totally scared. And excited. Can't believe it. In fact I can't sleep because of it. I'm worried about my Blazer too. Sgt. Perry came by late to see Jimmy, and brought me a bean bag dolphin like I almost got last week. It's so cute and it feels good to hold. Like it's got gel in it or something. It's a gorgeous shade of blue too. My ribs and chest is sore today. I've been crabby I know. My head hurts, but my chest is from the seat belt squeezing me. We figured that out when I went to Franklin. Now Sgt. Perry wants a plate with a Red Corvette on it (he collects vette stuff and we got him a blue one). Jimmy told him about the red one and now he wants one. We may go

get him one. They're only $1299 plus a plate holder for like a dollar. I told Jimmy we could get it from us if he wants to go get it. He's gonna make sure Sgt. Perry doesn't get one first. I'm glad the Sgt. likes it.

87. I got all my Current stuff. Talk about nice cards. They have really pretty ones. I'm glad I ordered a bunch. Jimmy says I'll never use all of the stuff I bought (because it's too cute and I'll save it I guess).

88. Got a 8x10 color picture autographed to me from Porter Waggoner today. Wonder how he knows I'm sick. It says get well soon. Oh and a note inside said get well and come back to the opry. I've been there once and met him. But no one really knows that. Anyway – apparantly my name is being passed around. Now maybe I should step it up and try to publish my book. Since I'm mingling with the Biggies of Nashville now. I can see me now --- a long beaded gown in a gorgeous color, new hair style and makeup. A Limo. Jimmy in a tux and the kids with diamond collars and professional shampoos and hairdo's. Dream on girl! I need to write Debbie. I forgot to have Mom call her. It saves me when she does that. Mom ordered me some Avon shower gel. Good stuff. I love it. That was so nice of her to do that. I'm glad she did. That stuff is so good. It leaves my skin soft and shiny. Even though its dry.

89. Well, it's bedtime and I just can't sleep. I should be tired, I took my pills (2) but I'm not sleepy. Jimmy started in on me at supper about everything. The dogs – he's fed up with them. All because Casey's rope is twisted after a few

days. So all dogs are pains in the butt ---- blah blah blah. Then he started in on how he wished he could be happy again. One day he will. And if I don't let him drive the Blazer I can pay the whole payment and cruise on down the road. He's got lots of girls who wants him. I never said I didn't. I did my hair different today. He never noticed 'till I mentioned it. Then he said it's ok. Later on he said he wasn't gonna get married again just live together. And I said not me. He snapped back that he REALLY DIDN'T CARE what I do anymore. Later he said I'm a prude and act like a nun. I dress like one too. Making fun of me. I asked him not to 'cause it hurts. I can't help how I look. I try to do the best I can every day. But I have some kind of medicine before bed and before I get up every morning plus every couple hours. It's hard on me dog gone it. I do good and try very hard. I don't whine and cry all the time. I just do what I can and try to be cheerful. All he see's is me being sick. Not the "trying" to cope or the cheerful part. That doesn't matter anymore. I'm serious now. He really wants me gone. He acts it, says it and I believe it. People ask him about me all the time because they like me and they care about me alot. Only I think it makes him jealous. He wanted to go to his folks Sun afternoon for steaks. Then he said we'd stay overnight and go see the doctor Mon. at 9:30 from there. I said NO. I'm not packing all my junk and leaving the kids that long. He knows that too. He wouldn't stay that long when I was in St. T's because of the dogs. Yet he said that to me. No way. He just wanted me to say no, so I could be the bad guy. I'm so tired of this game he plays. What will I do. I can't figure it out.

90. I'm scared I don't want to talk to Dan Marino. What if I get tongue tied? Or say something dumb. Why can't I just ask for a picture and autograph and say thanks. I love my Dolphins and wanna see them play in person. I'll make a short list that's what I'll do. Keep it simple. I tried another new hair style today. It really looks good too. Easy and fresh looking. Jimmy didn't notice. I hinted but he ignored it. This style is so cute. Like everyone is wearing. Parted on the side and behind the ears. The ends tuck under slightly. The rest is just natural. It looks softer and kind of romantic. I forgot my A.M. meds. today. I know I did. I feel it. But since I'm not positive (but I am) I just took 10 mgs. of steroids. That's all my body wants any more. I'm gonna go take aerosole and see if it helps. Until the 10 mgs kick in. It's a gorgeous day out. Spring is here finally. I hope it stays. I'm irrigating my nose more than 4 times a day. It helps with the blood clots. I'm hoping there aren't any on Mon. Then maybe I won't have to go back. Oh yuck I just thought of that nasty numbing stuff.

91. Went on a real date tonight. I looked good. Of course I was coughing by mid-date. I was so congested. But anyway, we went to K-Mart and Jimmy got this mower – I saw some hair stuff and almost got it. But we were going to Wal-Mart so I thought I'd check there. Jimmy mentioned that so I thought cool. We found it 5¢ cheaper, with a big bottle of shampoo and a bottle of creme rinse free! I mean it was too good. We got 3 of them. It's Citra-Shine. My books say it's good for adding shine to hair. My hair is a little dry looking. Not much but anyway this should

help. We ate at Burger King outside at a table under the stars. There was a gentle breeze and I kept wishing I was younger and then I'd be healthier. I know my shortness of breath is worse 'cause I forgot my prednisone. But it was so bad in Wal-Mart I was like, get me out of here and home. We saw our friend that manages Wal-Mart. She's so nice. She said she could tell I was having a hard time breathing. Thousands of dollars of meds. and aerosoles and I still can't breathe good. Will it ever get better (here on earth)? I want so bad to breathe good. I need air, oxygen or something. I try so hard to do everything right and I try to do things slow – still it's always the same. Wheezes, coughs, and gasps. I'm waiting for relief. Maybe in Florida. Someday.

92. Went to the nose doctor yesterday. Don't have to go back till I go see Dr. Haynes. (3 weeks.) Yea! Today we stayed around home and cleaned closets and finally decorated the TV thing so my Dan Marino and my dolphin plate would look good. Also my dolphin statutes. Now the whole TV stand looks good. Last night we got a call that said please wait for a very important message. 5 times it said that. Then I still waited about 2 minutes until it clicked off for some reason. I wonder if that was my call from Dan Marino and something happened to it. Jimmy says no – I think it was. Who knows. We went to Donna and Lynn's for a cookout Sun. A big ole steak and the works. It was so good. I enjoyed it. Then yesterday we ate out and today too. I'm full that's for sure. Jimmy mowed the whole yard already. Different parts at different times. But yesterday he did all of it. It took him 3 hours. But it looks good.

My Blazer is getting fixed too. We saw it today. Got a Bug shield and some anti-freeze for it. My poor Blazer. I love it so much. Can hardly wait for it to be fixed. I was squeeling and waiting as we pulled up to see it. We were talking about trying to go to Florida the first week in April. Only I can hardly ride to Franklin and back. I wheeze and choke so bad. I still have very little energy (if any) and I just cough so much I've had to increase my codeine. Instead of 3 or 4 a day I take like 6 or more some days. Others maybe 5. I really don't think I'll be able to go anywhere and have a good time. I'm too worn out and the mornings are real tough. Not only do I have to clear out but I have a stuffy nose till I wash it out and I have 2 aerosoles to do. It takes me a couple hours 'till I get all situated. That's why we couldn't stay with Donna and Lynn Sunday night. I told Jimmy I'm not into playing "sleep over" like kids do. It's just too much on me. Maybe later. Till then we'll have to keep on "keepin on"!

93. It's been a week or so since I've added on here. Alot's going on. I'm feeling better. But still tire easily and stay short of breath. Bad. Jimmy get's 4 days off next week. We were gonna go to Florida. Only our favorite place is booked up. Everything else is high. I'm way too worn out to go anyway. I can't clean house walk thru a store or anything without having a coughing spell. It's awful. I've found that my sleeping pills and pain pills were causing me to be short of breath too. Everything together was causing me problems. So now I know what to do to help a little anyway. Lee and Jenny left John they're out on their own again. Looking for a place. If I thought it'd work out Lee

could come and help me take care of my home and stuff 'till I get better. But I don't think it'd work out. With Jenny being a teenager and all. Everyone wanting to see TV and me wanting quiet plus I like my County CD's. Jen likes Rock. etc... It'd never work. I hope they do ok. Mom and Dad came by and we went out to eat chicken. I was asleep at first, but they surprised me. I'd been working on a tan and it had gotten cool and breezy so I came in the house. I'm getting a little brown so far. Just a tiny bit looks good on me 'cause I had no tan anymore from last year. Got McCaleb back. (My Blazer). He looks so good again. And we got Jimmy some bugle boy jeans and polo shirts from Goody's. He looks "fine" in them. I'll have to keep an eye peeled on him he looks so cute. Can't tell him that or he'll get all "ego tripped out" about it. He looks good and I don't. What a concept huh?

94. Got up today and for the first time my nose is clear feeling on both sides. I'm still having to irrigate it alot. I have to use antibiotic solution once a day too. It's alot of trouble to keep up with. I didn't know I'd have all this to do after nose surgery. Dr. Courey said something different before I had it done. He said I'd only need to irrigate for a couple weeks. Now it's everyday, forever. So I have to keep up with sterile water, and the med solution too. stuff! ok. Whatever. Some girl keeps calling here for Jimmy. He says it's a telemarketer. But she was giggling once. He doesn't know who it could be he says. But she sounds young. Did we get the groceries yesterday. Sixty dollars worth. That's with a bonus card. So it was maybe double that in value. What a difference Bi-Lo makes.

May 23rd

In St. T's again. Not for pneumonia or infection that's showing in the x-ray, anyways. It's my CF. I've got oxygen, morphine shots (every hour), steroids and a time release morphine pill too. It's all helping. I feel better. Dr. Haynes says I have 3 choices: lung transplant, pain meds. to keep me comfortable; or respirator. Which would mean lots of 24 hour extra care, and all that. I said pain meds. 'till I decide. I've gone down to 91 lbs! Talk about skin and bones, huh. Mom and Dad brought me in. Jimmy had a road block in Waynesboro, so anyway. Mom had stayed 2 nights so far.

May 30/June 1

This weeks' been so awful. First they couldn't cancel the vankomyacin.

Dear Jimmy,

I'm sitting on our deck – the breeze is blowing soft against my skin. It feels so good. Reminds me of when we were first married and we'd sleep with the window open. Or I'd be washing my hair in the bathtub at that white house, I'd raise up and the window was open. The breeze would blow the curtains and I could smell my shampoo. I was so happy. So in love. I never felt better.

Thank you for giving me such a beautiful life. You've always made sure I had what I wanted and needed. Plus extras! You've been good to me and loved me. Maybe more than I deserved at times. You're a good kind person. If I had my way you'd be so well rewarded for being the way you are. Of course you have your tough moments and we get on each other's nerves. But all in all I'd say we're a pretty good team.

I wish with all my heart that I could be the healthy beautiful "Babe" you deserve. It's not up to me though. But I do love you with every ounce of my being. I always have, and always will. I could never, ever have made it thru the hard times without you by my side. Never. You've been the one thing in this world I could always count on. You may not know it but I worship you. You are always on my mind. First in my thoughts above all else. I'm trying so hard to feel better. I want more good times. I want to be there for you when you need me. I want to tease you about stuff and make you crazy like I do sometimes. It's all a part of loving you. I know deep inside that you really love me. People have told me how you are when I'm not feeling good. How sad you are and stuff. You wouldn't be like that or put up with me if you didn't love me would you? No.

So I thought I'd write this down for you while I'm relaxing, and just say thanks for being you. And thanks for loving me so much. I'm gonna try real hard to get better. We've got things we want to do. Right? Most of all though – I just want to be with you wherever you are that's where I want to be. I'm lonely without my better half. So let's enjoy life more, and ease up on ourselves.

My wife Debbie of 16 years lost her battle with CF on June 9 at 5:53 AM. I had to watch her take her last breath while I was holding her hand. This is the day I lost my high school sweetheart which was the worst day of my life.

I would like to dedicate this book in her memory and all the ones with CF that are still battling this disease and for all the ones that have lost their fight and have gone to be with God.

Forgiveness

Bitterniss stunts growth,
pushes out God's love,
and locks the door
of communication;

But reconciliation
accelerates maturity
and lets love crawl back
through the open window
of humble hearts.

Mary Ann Cavender Hood